The Caregiver

and care

for the blind

MARTIN STERLING

Table of contents

Chapter 1: Understanding blindness — 13
Definition and classification of blindness — 14
Main causes of blindness — 14

- **Eye diseases**: glaucoma, cataracts, age-related macular degeneration (AMD), diabetic retinopathy. — 14

- **Neurological causes**: optic nerve damage, strokes affecting visual areas. — 17

- **Congenital and genetic causes**: abnormal eye development, hereditary diseases such as retinitis pigmentosa. — 23

Psychosocial impact of blindness — 29

Chapter 2: The caregiver's role with blind people — 35
Skills required — 36

- **Specific medical knowledge** — 36

- **Adapted communication skills** — 42

- **Empathy and patience** — 47

Ethics and deontology ... 52

Interprofessional collaboration ... 58

Chapter 3: Adapted communication techniques ... 65

Effective verbal communication ... 66

Body language and therapeutic touch ... 70

Use of assistive technologies ... 76

Chapter 4: Assistance with activities of daily living ... 83

Mobility and orientation ... 84

- Guiding techniques ... 84
- Travel safety ... 88
- Adapting to the environment ... 94

Personal care ... 101

Medication management ... 109

Chapter 5: Psychological and social support ... 117

Recognizing the signs of emotional distress ... 118

Psychological support techniques ... 123

Promoting social integration ... 129

Chapter 6: Rehabilitation and re-education ... 135

Vision rehabilitation programs ... 136

Learning Braille and other communication systems	142
Training for professional activities	149

Chapter 7: Legal aspects and available resources — 155

Rights of blind people	156
Support organizations and associations	161
Access to technology and financial aid	167

Chapter 8: Technological innovations in the care of blind people — 175

Modern devices and assistive technologies	176
• **Mobility aids**	176
○ Electronic rods	176
○ Customized GPS navigation systems	183
• **Voice and visual recognition technologies**	190
○ Screen reader applications	190
○ Object and text recognition software	198
• **Smart glasses and augmented reality**	205
Vision rehabilitation technologies	212

- Retinal implants and visual — 212
- Gene therapies and biomedical advances — 218
- Virtual reality in rehabilitation — 224

Integrating technology into daily care — 230

- Training nurses in the use of new technologies — 230
- Helping patients adopt technology — 232
- Data security and confidentiality — 236

Chapter 9: Integrating family and informal caregivers — 243

The family's role in the care process — 244

- Emotional and practical support — 244
- Collaboration with orderlies — 248

Communication and family education — 253

- Provide clear information on the patient's condition — 253
- Training relatives in assistance techniques — 256

Conflict management and family dynamics — 261

- Addressing disagreements about care — 261
- Support for families in distress — 267

Chapter 10: Specific care in a variety of environments — 275

Inpatient care — 276
- Specific protocols — 276
- Coordination with the medical team — 281

Care at home — 284
- Adapting the home environment — 284
- Planning visits and interventions — 290

Rehabilitation centers and specialized institutions — 297
- Intensive rehabilitation programs — 297

Chapter 11: Legislation and rights for blind people — 303

National and international legal framework — 304
- Accessibility and discrimination laws — 304
- International conventions (e.g. Convention on the Rights of Persons with Disabilities) — 309

Patient legal protection — 314
- Health rights — 314
- Remedies for rights violations — 320

The caregiver's role in advocacy — 326

- Patient awareness and education — 326
- Reporting abuse — 332

Chapter 12: Complementary and alternative approaches — 339

Sensory therapies — 340
- Music therapy — 340
- Aromatherapy — 344

Adapted physical activities — 348
- Yoga and meditation — 348
- Sports for the blind (goalball, judo) — 352

Art and creative expression — 359
- Plastic art workshops — 359
- Theater and oral expression — 363

Chapter 13: Emergency preparedness — 369

Appropriate first aid — 370
- Basic techniques — 370
- Crisis communication — 376

Evacuation and safety plans — 376
- Adapting emergency protocols — 376
- Training for exceptional situations (fires, natural disasters) — 381

Medical crisis management 387
- Recognizing warning signs 387
- Collaboration with emergency services 394

Chapter 14: The future of care for the blind 401

Emerging trends in healthcare 402
- Telemedicine and remote care 402
- Artificial intelligence and diagnostics 406

Patient participation in research 410
- Expert patient groups 410
- Co-construction of care protocols 415

Appendices 420
- Bibliographic resources 420

"Blindness is a condition that profoundly affects the daily lives of those who suffer from it. As a caregiver, your role is essential to ensure holistic care adapted to the specific needs of these patients. This book aims to provide you with the knowledge and tools you need to best support blind people, by combining medical theory and daily practice."

Chapter 1

Understanding blindness

Definition and classification of blindness

Blindness is defined as complete or partial loss of vision. It can be classified in different degrees, ranging from mild to total blindness. Understanding these classifications is essential for tailoring care to the patient's level of residual vision.

Main causes of blindness

- **Eye diseases**: glaucoma, cataracts, age-related macular degeneration (AMD), diabetic retinopathy.

Eye diseases :

Vision is an essential sense that enables us to interact with the world around us. Several eye pathologies can impair this ability, sometimes leading to blindness. Understanding these conditions is crucial for caregivers in adapting care and support to patients. Among the main eye pathologies responsible for blindness are glaucoma, cataracts, age-related macular degeneration (AMD) and diabetic retinopathy.

Glaucoma:

Glaucoma is a progressive optic neuropathy characterized by damage to the optic nerve, often associated with an increase in intraocular pressure (IOP). This rise in IOP generally results from an obstruction or malfunction of the system that evacuates the aqueous humor, the fluid that maintains pressure inside the eye.

The early stages of glaucoma are often asymptomatic, making early detection difficult. As the disease progresses, the patient may experience a progressive loss of peripheral visual field, evolving towards tunnel vision. Without proper treatment, glaucoma can lead to irreversible blindness.

Risk factors include advanced age, a family history of glaucoma, African origin, severe myopia and certain systemic diseases such as diabetes and hypertension. Treatment is aimed at reducing IOP to slow or halt disease progression, through hypotonizing eye drops, laser therapy or surgery.

For the caregiver, it's important to monitor compliance with medication, educate the patient on the importance of regular follow-ups, and recognize signs of worsening so that medical intervention can be prompt.

Cataracts :

Cataracts are characterized by the progressive opacification of the crystalline lens, the natural lens of the eye that focuses light on the retina. This opacification leads to reduced vision, increased sensitivity to bright light, halos around light sources and altered color perception.

Cataracts are mainly linked to aging, but other factors can also contribute to their development, such as eye trauma, prolonged exposure to ultraviolet rays, the use of certain medications (like corticosteroids) and metabolic diseases like diabetes.

The only effective treatment for cataracts is surgery. The opacified crystalline lens is removed and replaced by an artificial intraocular lens. This surgery is one of the most widely performed in the world, and generally offers a significant improvement in vision.

The caregiver's role is to accompany the patient before and after surgery. This includes pre-operative preparation, anxiety management, information on the operation and post-operative care such as administering eye drops, monitoring for signs of infection and educating on precautions for optimal recovery.

Age-related macular degeneration (AMD):

AMD is a degenerative condition that affects the macula, the central part of the retina responsible for fine vision and detail.

It is the leading cause of central vision loss in people over 50 in developed countries.

There are two forms of AMD:

- **The dry (atrophic) form**: characterized by progressive thinning of the macula, this form accounts for around 85% of cases. Loss of vision is slow and progressive.
- **The wet (neovascular) form**: less frequent but more severe, this is caused by the formation of abnormal blood vessels under the retina, leaking fluid or blood. Vision loss can be rapid and severe.

Symptoms include blurred vision, distortion of straight lines (metamorphopsia) and the appearance of a dark spot in the center of the visual field (central scotoma).

Risk factors include advanced age, smoking, genetic predisposition, a diet low in antioxidants and prolonged unprotected exposure to sunlight.

Treatment of wet AMD relies on intravitreal injections of anti-VEGF (vascular endothelial growth factor) to inhibit neovessel growth. Dry AMD has no curative treatment, but specific nutritional supplements can slow its progression.

Caregivers play a key role in supporting patients with AMD. They must encourage adherence to treatment, help manage daily activities affected by central vision loss, and provide psychological support in the face of the challenges posed by the disease.

Diabetic retinopathy :

Diabetic retinopathy is a microvascular complication of diabetes mellitus, resulting from chronic hyperglycemia that damages retinal blood vessels. It is a major cause of blindness in adults of working age.

The disease has two main stages:

- **Non-proliferative diabetic retinopathy**: characterized by microaneurysms, retinal hemorrhages and lipid exudates. At this stage, the patient may be asymptomatic or present with a slight reduction in visual acuity.
- **Proliferative diabetic retinopathy**: marked by the proliferation of fragile neovessels that can bleed into the vitreous, leading to more severe vision loss. Complications such as tractional retinal detachment can occur.

Symptoms include blurred vision, dark or empty areas in the visual field, and poor night vision.

Prevention and control of diabetic retinopathy rely on rigorous management of blood glucose, blood pressure and blood lipids. Treatments include laser photocoagulation to seal vascular leaks, intravitreal anti-VEGF injections and vitrectomy for persistent vitreous hemorrhage.

Caregivers play an essential role in the therapeutic education of diabetic patients. They must encourage self-management of the disease, promote compliance with treatment, monitor for signs of worsening, and coordinate care with other healthcare professionals.

- **Neurological causes**: optic nerve damage, strokes affecting visual areas.

Neurological causes :

Vision is the result of a complex process involving not only ocular structures, but also the central nervous system. Neurological damage can therefore lead to partial or total loss of vision, irrespective of the condition of the eyes themselves. Among these causes, optic nerve lesions and strokes affecting visual areas play a significant role. Understanding these mechanisms is essential for caregivers in order to offer appropriate support to the patients concerned.

Optic nerve damage :

The optic nerve is a crucial structure that transmits visual information from the retina to the brain. Damage to this nerve can lead to reduced visual acuity, alterations to the visual field and, in some cases, complete blindness in the affected eye.

Several conditions can damage the optic nerve:

1. **Optic neuritis:**
    Optic neuritis is an inflammation of the optic nerve, often associated with demyelinating diseases such as multiple sclerosis. Patients generally present with a sudden, painful loss of vision in one eye, sometimes accompanied by disturbances in color perception (dyschromatopsia).
    Diagnosis is based on ophthalmological examination, measurement of visual acuity and visual field, and complementary tests such as magnetic resonance imaging (MRI). Treatment consists of corticosteroids to reduce inflammation, and management of the underlying disease.

2. **Anterior ischemic optic neuropathy:**
    This condition results from an interruption of blood flow in the arteries supplying the optic nerve head. It often occurs in elderly patients with vascular risk factors such as hypertension, diabetes and hypercholesterolemia.
    Symptoms include painless, usually unilateral, vision loss and visual field defects. Management is aimed at controlling cardiovascular risk factors to prevent recurrence.

3. **Optic nerve compression**:
   Intracranial masses such as tumors (meningiomas, gliomas), aneurysms or cysts can compress the optic nerve, leading to progressive vision loss. Signs may include headaches, visual field abnormalities and sometimes hormonal disturbances if the pituitary region is involved.
   Diagnosis is based on brain imaging (MRI, CT scan), and treatment may involve surgery, radiotherapy or chemotherapy, depending on the nature of the lesion.

4. **Head trauma**:
   Trauma to the orbit or skull can damage the optic nerve. Vision loss may be immediate or delayed, depending on the mechanism of injury. Treatment is often urgent and multidisciplinary, involving neurosurgeons and ophthalmologists.

5. **Toxic and deficiency-induced optic neuropathies**:
   Exposure to certain toxic substances (methanol, ethambutol) or nutritional deficiencies (vitamin B12 deficiency) can affect the optic nerve. Patients experience progressive bilateral vision loss and abnormal color vision.
   Treatment consists of eliminating exposure to the toxin or correcting the deficiency, with visual recovery varying according to the speed of intervention.

The role of the caregiver in optic nerve damage :

The caregiver must be alert to signs of visual deterioration in at-risk patients, such as those with multiple sclerosis or vascular risk factors. He or she helps ensure compliance with treatment, educates patients about the importance of medical follow-up, and provides psychological support in the face of visual loss.

Strokes affecting visual areas :

Stroke can affect brain regions involved in visual perception, leading to specific deficits depending on the location of the lesion.

1. **Anatomy of the visual pathways:**
   Visual information captured by the retina is transmitted via the optic nerve, the optic chiasm, the optic tracts, the lateral geniculate body of the thalamus, then the optic radiations to the primary visual cortex located in the occipital lobe.

2. **Occipital lobe stroke:**
   Ischemia or hemorrhage in the occipital lobe can lead to cortical blindness, where the patient is blind despite having functional eyes. Patients may not recognize their blindness (Anton's syndrome) and pretend to see normally.
   Symptoms include bilateral vision loss, visual hallucinations and difficulty interpreting visual information.

3. **Homonymous hemianopsia:**
   If the stroke affects the optic radiations or visual cortex unilaterally, the patient may experience homonymous hemianopsia, i.e. a loss of half the visual field on the same side in both eyes.
   This can lead to difficulties in daily activities, such as bumping into objects on the affected side, or overlooking people or food on that side.

4. **Quadranopsia:**
   More localized lesions can cause a loss of a quarter of the visual field (quadranopsia), affecting the ability to read, recognize faces or navigate the environment.

The caregiver's role in stroke affecting vision :

Caregivers need to be trained to recognize the signs of a stroke so that they can take prompt action, which is crucial to limiting neurological damage. After the stroke, the role involves :

- **Assess visual deficits**: work with the medical team to determine the extent of losses and adapt care accordingly.
- **Adapting the environment**: organizing the patient's living space to minimize obstacles, placing important objects on the unaffected side.
- **Stimulate visual rehabilitation**: encourage exercises prescribed by specialists to recover or compensate for deficits.
- **Assisting with daily activities**: helping with eating, mobility and hygiene, while promoting independence whenever possible.
- **Psychological support**: patients may experience frustration, anxiety or depression in the face of sudden vision loss. Empathic listening and emotional support are essential.

Other neurological disorders affecting vision :

1. **Demyelinating diseases:**
   In addition to multiple sclerosis, other demyelinating diseases can affect the visual pathways, such as neuromyelitis optica (Devic's disease), which causes severe optic neuritis that is often bilateral.

2. **Toxic or metabolic encephalopathies:**
   Metabolic disorders (Wernicke's encephalopathy due to thiamine deficiency) or exposure to toxins can impair cortical visual functions.

3. **Occipital epilepsy:**
   Focused epileptic seizures in the occipital lobe may cause visual hallucinations or temporary loss of vision.

4. **Migraine with visual aura:**
   Some migraines are accompanied by transient visual phenomena, such as flickering scotomas, zigzag lines or temporary hemianopsia.

The importance of understanding neurological causes :

For the caregiver, it is essential to understand that vision loss can result from impairments beyond the eye. This influences the approach to care, as the patient's needs can be complex, involving associated motor, cognitive or sensory deficits. Close collaboration with neurologists, ophthalmologists, orthoptists and occupational therapists is necessary to develop a comprehensive care plan.

Holistic approach to care :

1. **Multidisciplinary assessment:**
   Participate in consultation meetings to understand diagnosis, prognosis and treatment goals.

2. **Adapted communication :**
   Use appropriate communication techniques, taking into account possible language (aphasia) or comprehension disorders.

3. **Promoting autonomy:**
   Encourage patients to take an active part in their rehabilitation, valuing their progress and setting realistic goals.

4. **Continuing education:**
   Keep abreast of advances in the management of visual neurological disorders, by attending specific training courses.

- **Congenital and genetic causes**: abnormal eye development, hereditary diseases such as retinitis pigmentosa.

Congenital and genetic causes :

Blindness can be the result of conditions present from birth or passed on genetically. These conditions profoundly affect the development of the individual and his or her interaction with the surrounding world. Understanding these causes is essential for the caregiver, as they require specific management, family support and long-term care planning. Among the main congenital and genetic causes of blindness are anomalies in eye development and hereditary diseases such as retinitis pigmentosa.

Eye development abnormalities :

Ocular development anomalies are defects occurring during gestation, affecting the normal formation of eye structures. These anomalies may be isolated or associated with more complex syndromes involving other organ systems.

1. **Anophthalmos and microphthalmos:**
    - **Anophthalmos**: complete absence of the eye. This rare condition can be unilateral or bilateral, resulting from an early interruption in the embryonic development of the eye.
    - **Microphthalmia**: reduction in the size of the eye, making it abnormally small. The degree of residual vision depends on the severity of the malformation.
2. These anomalies can be caused by genetic mutations, maternal infections (such as rubella), or exposure to teratogenic toxins or drugs during pregnancy.

3. **Coloboma:**
   A coloboma is a fissure or absence of tissue in part of the eye, resulting from incomplete closure of the embryonic optic cleft. It can affect the iris, retina, choroid or optic nerve, resulting in variable visual deficits depending on the location and extent of the lesion.

4. **Congenital cataract:**
   A congenital cataract is an opacification of the crystalline lens present from birth or appearing in early childhood. It can be unilateral or bilateral, and seriously compromises the development of vision if not treated promptly.
   Causes include genetic mutations, intrauterine infections (toxoplasmosis, rubella, cytomegalovirus), metabolic diseases (such as galactosemia) or genetic syndromes. Treatment consists of early surgical removal of the opacified lens, followed by appropriate optical correction.

5. **Congenital glaucoma :**
   Congenital glaucoma is a rare disease characterized by elevated intraocular pressure due to an abnormality in the development of aqueous humor drainage structures. Symptoms include corneal enlargement (buphthalmia), tearing, photophobia and corneal opacification.
   Treatment is surgical and must be carried out rapidly to preserve vision. Long-term follow-up is essential, as further interventions may be necessary.

6. **Ocular albinism:**
   Albinism is a genetic condition characterized by reduced or absent production of melanin, the pigment that gives skin, hair and eyes their color. In ocular albinism, patients present with hypopigmentation of the iris and retina, resulting in sensitivity to light,

nystagmus (involuntary eye movements) and poor visual acuity.

Hereditary diseases :

Hereditary diseases affecting vision are due to genetic mutations passed down from generation to generation. They can affect different structures of the eye or visual pathways, leading to progressive vision loss.

1. **Retinitis pigmentosa :**
   Retinitis pigmentosa is a group of hereditary retinal dystrophies characterized by progressive degeneration of the photoreceptors, mainly rods and then cones. Patients experience night blindness (nyctalopia), a reduction in the peripheral visual field (tunnel vision) and, at an advanced stage, a reduction in central visual acuity.
   The disease can be inherited in different ways: autosomal dominant, autosomal recessive or X-linked. There is great variability in the age of onset and progression of the disease. There is currently no cure, but research is underway into gene therapy and retinal implants.

2. **Leber's congenital amaurosis:**
   This is a severe form of retinal dystrophy present from birth or early childhood, leading to blindness or very poor vision. Patients may experience nystagmus, photophobia and delayed motor development as a result of the visual impairment.
   Gene therapies have shown promising results for some genetic subtypes of the disease, improving visual function in some patients.

3. **Stargardt's disease:**
   Stargardt's disease is an inherited macular dystrophy that causes progressive loss of central vision. It usually

appears in childhood or adolescence. Patients have difficulty reading and recognizing faces, and may have impaired color vision.

There is no cure, but clinical trials are exploring potential treatment options. Protection from intense light is recommended to slow disease progression.

4. **Leber's hereditary optic neuropathy:**
This is a mitochondrial disease transmitted through the mother, mainly affecting young men. It is characterized by a sudden, painless loss of central vision in one eye, followed by the other eye within a few weeks or months.

Management is mainly symptomatic, with research underway into treatments aimed at improving mitochondrial function.

Role of the caregiver in congenital and genetic causes :

Caring for patients with congenital or genetic blindness requires a holistic approach centered on the patient and his or her family. The caregiver plays an essential role in :

1. **Supporting children's development :**

   - **Sensory stimulation**: Encourage the use of other senses (touch, hearing, smell) to promote cognitive and motor development.

   - **Adapting activities**: Offer adapted games and exercises to stimulate learning and independence.

2. **Family support :**

   - **Information and education**: Provide clear information on the child's condition, care options and available resources.

- **Emotional support**: listening to parents' concerns, helping them overcome the shock of the diagnosis and adapt to the situation.

3. **Care coordination :**

    - **Multidisciplinary teamwork**: Collaborate with ophthalmologists, orthoptists, occupational therapists, psychologists and specialist teachers to develop a comprehensive care plan.

    - **Treatment and rehabilitation follow-up**: Ensure continuity of care, monitor treatment compliance and participate in rehabilitation sessions.

4. **Promoting social integration :**

    - **Inclusive education**: Supporting the child's integration into adapted or mainstream school structures, with the necessary accommodations.

    - **Social and recreational activities**: Encourage participation in sports, artistic and cultural activities to foster personal fulfillment.

5. **Preparing for independence :**

    - **Teaching daily living skills**: Helping children learn to move around independently, dress themselves, feed themselves and communicate effectively.

    - **Use of assistive technologies**: Familiarize patients with technical aids such as audio playback devices, adapted software and Braille.

6. **Psychological support :**

      ◦ **Managing emotions**: Help children and families express their feelings and develop positive coping strategies.

      ◦ **Isolation prevention**: Encourage social interaction and participation in support groups or patient associations.

Importance of early detection :

Early detection and intervention are crucial to maximizing the developmental potential of children with congenital or genetic visual impairments. The caregiver must be alert to signs of visual impairment in newborns and young children, such as lack of visual tracking, nystagmus, or maladaptive response to light stimuli.

In case of suspicion, it is essential to refer the child rapidly to a pediatric ophthalmologist for a thorough evaluation. Early referral to a pediatric ophthalmologist enables the initiation of appropriate interventions, such as vision rehabilitation, and optimizes the child's chances of development.

Ethical and respectful approach:

It is important to consider the emotional and social impact of congenital and genetic disorders on the patient and his or her family. The caregiver must adopt an empathetic attitude, respecting the patient's dignity and choices, and avoiding judgment or prejudice. It is also essential to respect confidentiality and support the patient's autonomy wherever possible.

News and outlook :

Advances in medical genetics offer new prospects for diagnosis, genetic counseling and the development of innovative therapies. Gene therapies, stem cells and retinal prostheses are promising areas of research that could transform the management of these diseases in the future.

Caregivers need to keep abreast of these developments to advise patients on emerging possibilities, direct them to clinical trials where appropriate, and adapt their practice accordingly.

Psychosocial impact of blindness

Blindness, whether congenital or acquired, has profound repercussions on the lives of those affected. Beyond sensory loss, it significantly affects psychological well-being, self-esteem, social relationships and participation in community life. Understanding this psychosocial impact is essential for caregivers, as it enables them to adapt their support and promote a better quality of life for patients.

Psychological reactions to vision loss

Vision loss, especially when acquired, is often experienced as a major trauma. Patients may go through various emotional phases similar to the stages of grief described by Elisabeth Kübler-Ross:

1. **Shock and denial**: When the diagnosis is announced, some patients refuse to believe in the reality of their condition. This temporary defense mechanism protects them from the unbearable anguish of blindness.

2. **Anger**: Once reality has been accepted, frustration and anger may emerge. The patient may feel unjustly treated by fate, and feel rage against healthcare professionals, family or themselves.

3. **Bargaining**: the patient seeks solutions to regain lost vision, sometimes clinging to unproven treatments or increasing the number of medical consultations.

4. **Depression**: Faced with the irreversibility of their condition, patients can fall into a state of depression, characterized by profound sadness, loss of interest in usual activities, sleep and appetite disturbances, and even suicidal thoughts.

5. **Acceptance**: With time and the right support, patients can come to terms with their situation, enabling a positive adjustment and the development of new life projects.

Impact on self-esteem and identity

Vision plays a central role in self-perception and interaction with the environment. Blindness can alter the patient's self-image, leading to a drop in self-esteem. Feelings of uselessness, dependence and incompetence can set in, especially if the patient is forced to abandon previously rewarding professional or personal activities.

Redefining identity is a complex process that takes time. Patients must integrate their visual impairment into their self-perception, without reducing themselves to it. The caregiver can play a key role by valuing the patient's remaining skills, encouraging him or her to develop new abilities, and recognizing his or her efforts and achievements.

Social isolation and stigmatization

Blindness can lead to withdrawal and social isolation. Physical and environmental obstacles, such as the inaccessibility of public places or transport, limit the patient's participation in social activities. In addition, the fear of endangering oneself or depending on others can discourage the patient from leaving home.

The stigma and prejudice associated with blindness exacerbate this isolation. Blind people are sometimes perceived as incapable, which can lead to paternalistic or discriminatory attitudes on the part of society. These negative experiences reinforce the feeling of exclusion and can lead to self-stigmatization, where the patient integrates these devaluing beliefs.

Impact on family and professional relationships

Blindness changes family dynamics. Relatives may become anxious, frustrated or tired when faced with new responsibilities. Sometimes, overprotection can set in, limiting the patient's autonomy and generating tensions. It is essential to encourage open communication within the family, so that everyone's needs and feelings can be expressed.

At work, vision loss may force the patient to quit or change jobs. This entails not only financial loss, but also a loss of professional identity and the social network associated with work. Vocational retraining or adaptation of the workstation are major issues in maintaining the patient's inclusion in the world of work.

Adaptation strategies and resilience

Despite these challenges, many patients develop effective coping strategies that enable them to lead fulfilling lives. These include:

- **Active acceptance**: Rather than denying or fighting the reality of blindness, the patient chooses to integrate it into their life and focus on what they can control.

- **Finding social support**: Surrounding yourself with understanding and caring people, joining support groups or associations for blind people can bring comfort and practical advice.

- **Developing new skills**: Learning Braille, using assistive technology, or engaging in new activities can restore a sense of mastery and independence.

- **Positive reappraisal**: Some patients manage to find meaning in their experience, developing a new philosophy of life or getting involved in causes close to their hearts.

The caregiver's role in psychosocial support

The caregiver is in a privileged position to support the patient in this adaptation process. Here's how he can help:

1. **Empathetic listening**: offering an attentive, non-judgmental presence, allowing the patient to express his or her emotions and concerns. The caregiver must recognize the legitimacy of the patient's feelings and avoid minimizing his or her suffering.

2. **Information and education**: Providing clear information about blindness, available resources, technical aids and possible adaptations. A better understanding of the condition helps patients regain control over their lives.

3. **Promoting autonomy**: Encouraging patients to carry out the activities they are capable of doing themselves. Learning mobility techniques, how to manage daily tasks and the use of appropriate tools helps to boost self-confidence.

4. **Support for social and professional reintegration**: Help patients identify training, leisure and employment opportunities suited to their situation. Collaborate with specialized services to facilitate reintegration.

5. **Management of psychological disorders**: Identify signs of depression, anxiety or post-traumatic stress. Refer patients to mental health professionals if necessary, while continuing to provide day-to-day support.

6. **Raising awareness**: Work with family and friends to foster mutual understanding. Explain the importance of the patient's autonomy and how they can support him without overprotecting him.

7. **Adapting the environment**: Participating in the design of the patient's living space to make it safe and accessible. This includes organizing personal items, removing obstacles and using tactile or acoustic cues.

The importance of appropriate communication

Communication is a key element in psychosocial support. The caregiver must adopt appropriate communication techniques:

- **Physical presence**: Position yourself in front of the patient, informing him of your presence and actions to avoid surprising him.

- **Use of clear language**: Avoid visual expressions such as "look here" or "you see". Use precise, detailed descriptions.

- **Continuous feedback**: Regularly check the patient's comprehension, paying attention to verbal and non-verbal reactions.

- **Patience and respect for rhythm**: Allow patients to express themselves at their own pace, without rushing or interrupting them.

Promoting social inclusion

The caregiver can encourage the patient to maintain or develop social ties:

- **Participation in group activities**: Offer workshops, cultural outings or adapted sports activities.

- **Community involvement**: Encourage patients to get involved in associations, support groups or volunteer work.

- **Use of technology**: Familiarize patients with modern communication tools, such as adapted smartphones, social networks or voice messaging applications.

Preventing digital isolation

In an increasingly connected society, access to online information and services is essential. Blindness can be a barrier to this access if the patient is not trained in the appropriate technologies. The caregiver can :

- **Train patients to use screen readers**: these software programs transform text displayed on the screen into speech synthesis or tactile Braille.

- **Present accessible applications and websites**: Help patients navigate the Internet, use online banking services, communication platforms or health management tools.

- **Ensuring digital security**: making patients aware of the risks associated with using the Internet and how to protect their personal data.

Chapter 2

The caregiver's role with blind people

Skills required

- **Specific medical knowledge**

The effective care of blind people requires a thorough command of specific medical knowledge. This knowledge encompasses a detailed understanding of the anatomy and physiology of the eye, the various pathologies leading to blindness, and the treatments and interventions available. It also includes familiarity with assistive technologies, the principles of rehabilitation, and the legal aspects of visual impairment. This medical expertise is essential for providing appropriate care, anticipating potential complications and accompanying patients through their health care journey.

Anatomy and physiology of the eye and visual system

Understanding the structure and function of the eye is fundamental to understanding the mechanisms of visual impairment. The eye is a complex organ made up of several key structures:

- **The cornea**: The eye's first lens, it helps focus light.
- **The iris and pupil**: regulate the amount of light entering the eye.
- **The crystalline lens**: Biconvex lens that adjusts focus for sharp vision at different distances.
- **Retina**: Nerve tissue containing photoreceptors (rods and cones) responsible for converting light into electrical signals.
- **The optic nerve**: transmits visual signals from the retina to the brain's visual cortex.

Understanding these structures and their interrelationships enables the caregiver to grasp how different pathologies affect vision.

Main pathologies leading to blindness

1. **Glaucoma**: A disease characterized by elevated intraocular pressure, leading to optic neuropathy and progressive loss of peripheral visual field. Glaucoma is often asymptomatic in its early stages, making early detection crucial. Treatments aim to reduce intraocular pressure by means of hypotensive eye drops, laser or surgical interventions.

2. **Cataract**: Progressive opacification of the crystalline lens, leading to reduced visual acuity, increased sensitivity to glare and impaired color perception. Treatment is surgical, replacing the opacified crystalline lens with an artificial intraocular lens.

3. **Age-related macular degeneration (AMD)**: Degenerative disease of the macula, responsible for central vision and fine detail. AMD can be dry (atrophic) or wet (neovascular). Treatments include intravitreal anti-VEGF injections for the wet form and nutritional supplements for the dry form.

4. **Diabetic retinopathy**: A microvascular complication of diabetes, characterized by damage to retinal blood vessels. It can lead to retinal hemorrhages, exudates and, ultimately, retinal detachment. Prevention is based on strict control of blood sugar levels and cardiovascular risk factors. Treatments include laser photocoagulation and intravitreal injections.

5. **Neurological damage**: Damage to the optic nerve, such as optic neuritis, or strokes affecting the visual areas can lead to vision loss. Management depends on the underlying cause, and may include immunomodulatory treatments or visual rehabilitation.

6. **Hereditary diseases**: genetic disorders such as retinitis pigmentosa cause progressive degeneration of

photoreceptors, leading to loss of night and peripheral vision. Treatment options are limited, but research is underway into gene therapy.

Symptoms and clinical signs to recognize

The caregiver must be alert to clinical signs of impaired visual function:

- **Decreased visual acuity**: difficulty reading, recognizing faces or seeing at a distance.
- **Impaired visual field**: tunnel vision, blind spots, difficulty perceiving objects to the side.
- **Photophobia**: Excessive sensitivity to light.
- **Diplopia**: Double vision.
- **Eye pain**: may indicate inflammation or increased intraocular pressure.
- **Nystagmus**: Rapid involuntary eye movements.

Recognizing these signs can quickly alert the medical team for appropriate treatment.

Principles of treatment and intervention

Knowledge of available treatments is essential to support the patient:

- **Drug treatments**: administration of eye drops, ocular antihypertensives, anti-inflammatories.
- **Surgical procedures**: Cataract surgery, trabeculectomy for glaucoma, vitrectomy.
- **Laser therapies**: Used to treat diabetic retinopathy or AMD.
- **Visual rehabilitation**: Personalized programs to optimize the use of residual vision.

The caregiver is responsible for ensuring patient compliance, explaining treatment procedures and monitoring side effects.

Assistive technologies and visual aids

Familiarity with assistive technologies is crucial to promoting patient autonomy:

- **Optical aids**: magnifiers, wide-field glasses.
- **Electronic devices**: screen readers, text-to-speech software, mobile applications for the blind.
- **Mobility aids**: White cane, electronic guidance devices.
- **Braille**: Tactile writing system for reading and communication.

The caregiver must be able to advise the patient on the options available and help him or her learn how to use them.

Principles of rehabilitation and re-education

Rehabilitation aims to help the patient develop skills to compensate for vision loss:

- **Orientation and mobility**: Techniques for getting around safely, using auditory and tactile cues.
- **Activities of daily living**: Adapting methods for personal hygiene, meal preparation and household management.
- **Communication**: Braille learning, use of adapted communication technologies.
- **Psychological support**: Help in coping with the emotional challenges of blindness.

The caregiver works with occupational therapists, orthoptists and other professionals to set up an appropriate rehabilitation plan.

Legal and ethical aspects

Knowledge of the rights of blind people is essential:

- **Accessibility**: Knowledge of legal standards for the accessibility of buildings, transport and services.

- **Financial aid**: Information on grants, subsidies and financial support schemes.
- **Discrimination**: Raising awareness of laws protecting against discrimination in the workplace, education and public services.
- **Confidentiality**: Respect for patients' personal and medical data.

Caregivers must defend patients' interests, advise them on their rights and ensure that the care they receive is ethical.

Comorbidities and associated complications

Blind patients may have comorbidities that influence their management:

- **Diabetes**: Requires regular monitoring of blood sugar levels, nutritional management and prevention of complications.
- **Hypertension**: Blood pressure control to reduce cardiovascular and ocular risks.
- **Neurological disorders**: Monitoring of neurological symptoms, coordination with neurologists.
- **Mental health**: Screening for depression and anxiety, referral to professionals if necessary.

The caregiver must adopt a holistic approach, taking into account all the patient's needs.

Appropriate communication with the patient

Effective communication is the key to building trust:

- **Clear, precise language**: avoid ambiguous terms, describe actions performed.
- **Pay attention to non-verbal cues**: Even if the patient can't see, tone of voice, rhythm and volume are important.

- **Respect and patience**: Take the time to listen, respect the patient's rhythm, don't rush him or her.
- **Continuous information**: Explain each stage of care, ensuring patient understanding.

This communication promotes patient autonomy and involvement in care.

Updating knowledge and continuing education

The medical field is constantly evolving. The nursing auxiliary must engage in continuous training in order to :

- **Keep abreast of therapeutic advances**: new molecules, innovative technologies, updated protocols.
- **Participate in specialized training**: Workshops, seminars, conferences on blindness and related care.
- **Exchange with peers**: share experiences, best practices and challenges.
- **Contribute to improving care**: Participate in research projects, quality audits, professional practice committees.

This approach enables us to offer high-quality care and to innovate in daily practice.

Psychological and social support

Understanding the psychosocial impact of blindness is crucial:

- **Emotional support**: helping patients to express their feelings, supporting them in their adaptation phases.
- **Isolation prevention**: Encourage social interaction and participation in community activities.
- **Referral to resources**: support groups, patient associations, social services.
- **Family involvement**: Working with family members to support the patient, providing information and advice.

The caregiver thus contributes to the patient's overall well-being.

- **Adapted communication skills**

Adapted communication skills

Communication is an essential pillar in the relationship between the caregiver and the blind patient. It goes far beyond the simple transmission of medical information; it encompasses the establishment of a relationship of trust, emotional support and the promotion of the patient's autonomy. Developing appropriate communication skills is therefore fundamental to meeting the specific needs of blind people and ensuring quality care.

The importance of appropriate communication

The loss of vision profoundly alters the way a person interacts with their environment. Blind patients rely more heavily on their other senses, particularly hearing and touch, to understand their surroundings. Clear, precise verbal communication is therefore essential. Not only does it convey essential information, it also reassures the patient, prevents misunderstandings and promotes psychological well-being.

Fundamentals of communication with blind patients

1. **Introduce yourself clearly and announce your presence**
   During every interaction, it's important to introduce yourself by giving your name and job title. For example: "Hello Mr. Martin, I'm Sophie, your care assistant. This lets the patient know who he or she is talking to, and avoids any confusion or anxiety linked to an unexpected presence.

2. **Explaining future actions**
   Before taking any action, it's essential to inform the

patient of what you're going to do. For example: "I'm now going to check your blood pressure by placing the cuff on your left arm." This reassures the patient and prepares him or her mentally for the procedure.

3. **Use clear, precise language** Avoid vague or ambiguous expressions. Give preference to detailed descriptions using spatial cues. For example, rather than saying "It's this way", specify "The bathroom door is on your right, three steps ahead."

4. **Adapt tone and rhythm of speech**
Speak clearly, at a moderate pace, with good articulation. It is not necessary to speak louder, unless the patient also has a hearing impairment. Your intonation should be warm and respectful.

5. **Avoiding purely visual gestures and expressions**
Blind patients cannot perceive facial expressions or hand gestures. So it's important to translate these non-verbal signals into words. For example, instead of nodding your head in approval, express your agreement verbally.

Specific techniques for effective communication

1. **Active listening**
Show the patient that you are fully attentive to what he or she is saying. This means letting them express themselves without interruption, rephrasing their words to confirm your understanding, and asking open-ended questions to probe certain points. For example: "Can you tell me how you feel today?"

2. **Empathy**
Put yourself in the patient's shoes to understand their emotions and concerns. Express your understanding with phrases like "I understand how frustrating this can

be for you" or "This must be difficult to deal with, I'm here to help."

3. **Respecting the patient's rhythm**
   Everyone communicates at their own pace. Give patients time to formulate their thoughts, without rushing them. Be patient and avoid completing sentences for them.

4. **Appropriate use of touch**
   Touch can be a powerful means of communication and comfort, but it must be used with sensitivity and consent. Always ask permission before touching the patient. For example, "May I take your arm to guide you to your chair?"

5. **Consistency and constancy**
   Try to maintain routines in your interactions. Blind patients can find comfort in predictability. Inform them in advance of any changes in schedules or routine procedures.

Avoid clumsiness and stereotypes

Some common expressions may be inappropriate. For example, avoid saying "Look" or "See", even though these expressions are often used figuratively. Instead, use terms like "Listen", "Let me explain", or "Do you understand?". Also, avoid making assumptions about a patient's abilities or limitations based on their blindness. Each person is unique, with his or her own skills and needs.

Facilitating spatial orientation

Helping patients find their way around is crucial. Give clear directions using precise landmarks. For example:

- **Directional indications**: Use points of the compass (north, south, east, west) or time markers ("The table is at 3 o'clock").
- **Description of environment**: Detail furniture layout, presence of obstacles or changes in floor surface.
- **Physical guidance**: If you are guiding the patient, let him hold your arm rather than pulling or pushing him. Walk slightly ahead of him, informing him of changes in direction or obstacles.

Encouraging autonomy and participation

Involving patients in decisions about their care promotes their autonomy and self-esteem. Ask them about their preferences and respect their choices. For example, "Do you prefer to shower now or after breakfast? Encourage them to carry out the tasks they are capable of doing themselves, offering your assistance if necessary.

Use of assistive technologies

Familiarize yourself with technological tools that can facilitate communication and patient autonomy:

- **Text-to-speech devices**: Enable patients to access written information, such as menus, appointment schedules or medical instructions.
- **Adapted mobile applications**: help with navigation, object recognition and medication management.
- **Braille reading devices**: For patients who have mastered Braille, these devices can be invaluable for written communication.

By understanding these tools, you can better support your patients in using them and integrate them into their daily care.

Communication in group situations

When a blind patient is present in a group, for example at group activities or family gatherings, it is important to include him or her actively:

- **Introduce those present**: Indicate who is in the room, specifying their relative position.
- **Facilitate interactions**: Encourage others to speak directly to the patient and follow the same principles of adapted communication.
- **Avoid multiple simultaneous conversations**: Criss-crossing exchanges can be difficult for the patient to follow.

Managing emotions and stress

Blindness can be a source of anxiety, frustration and sadness. Appropriate communication can provide emotional support:

- **Acknowledge his feelings**: Show that you are attentive to his emotional state. For example, "You seem preoccupied today, would you like to talk about it?"
- **Offer support**: Offer your help in finding solutions to the problems they encounter.
- **Respect the patient's privacy**: If the patient doesn't want to discuss certain topics, respect his or her choice.

Ongoing training and self-assessment

Improving your communication skills is an ongoing process. Don't hesitate to :

- **Participate in specialized training**: Workshops on communicating with blind people can enrich your practices.

- **Ask for feedback**: Solicit the patient's opinion on the way you communicate. It shows your commitment and helps you adapt.
- **Observe experienced colleagues**: Learn the approaches and techniques used by other professionals.

- **Empathy and patience**

When caring for blind people, empathy and patience are essential qualities that caregivers must cultivate to offer quality care and promote the patient's well-being. These two interpersonal skills make it possible to create a relationship of trust, accompany patients in their daily challenges and support their autonomy and social integration.

Empathy: understanding and sharing the patient's feelings

Empathy is the ability to put oneself in another person's shoes, to understand their emotions, needs and experiences without judging them. For the caregiver, this implies :

- **Recognizing the patient's emotions**: Blind people can experience complex feelings such as frustration, fear, anxiety or sadness. By being aware of these emotions, caregivers can better adapt their approach and support.

- **Emotional support**: Empathy provides reassurance, comfort and encouragement. It fosters open communication in which the patient feels listened to and understood.

- **Tailoring care to individual needs**: Every patient is unique. By understanding their preferences, values and goals, caregivers can tailor interventions to be truly beneficial.

- **Promoting autonomy**: By recognizing patients' abilities and resources, caregivers can encourage them to participate actively in their care and develop new skills.

Patience: accompanying patients at their own pace

Patience is the ability to tolerate delays, obstacles or difficulties without becoming overwhelmed by frustration or impatience. In the context of caring for blind people, patience is demonstrated by :

- **Respect the time needed**: Some tasks or learning may take longer for a blind person. The caregiver must be prepared to repeat information, explain calmly and wait until the patient feels ready.

- **Dealing with frustration**: Patients may express irritation or anger at their situation. Patience enables us to remain calm, not to take these reactions personally, and to continue to offer sympathetic support.

- **Encourage gradually**: Patience is essential to help patients overcome their fears and hesitations. By taking things one step at a time, the caregiver facilitates learning and builds the patient's confidence.

How to integrate empathy and patience into daily practice

1. **Attentive listening**
   Take the time to listen to the patient without interrupting, showing genuine interest in what he or she is saying. Active listening involves rephrasing the

patient's words to ensure you understand his or her needs.

2. **Non-verbal observation**
   Even if the patient is blind, he may express his emotions through his tone of voice, posture or gestures. Paying attention to these signals helps us to better understand the patient's emotional state.

3. **Clear, reassuring communication**
   Use simple language, avoid medical jargon, and explain each stage of care. Informing the patient of what's to come reduces anxiety and boosts confidence.

4. **Adapting to patient reactions**
   If the patient becomes frustrated or agitated, remain calm and understanding. Offer a break if necessary, and resume activities when he/she feels ready.

5. **Encouragement and recognition**
   Recognize patients' efforts and progress, even the smallest ones, to boost motivation and self-esteem.

The benefits of empathy and patience for both patient and caregiver

- **Strengthening the therapeutic relationship**: A relationship based on trust and mutual understanding facilitates collaboration and improves the effectiveness of care.

- **Improved patient well-being**: Empathetic, patient support helps patients manage stress, reduce anxiety and increase satisfaction with the care they receive.

- **Preventing burnout**: For the caregiver, adopting an empathetic and patient attitude contributes to better stress management and increased job satisfaction.

Challenges and obstacles to overcome

It's important to recognize that practicing empathy and patience can be challenging:

- **Occupational stress**: Time constraints, workloads and complex situations can put the caregiver's patience to the test.

- **Personal emotions**: Caregivers may experience their own emotions, such as fatigue or frustration, which can influence their ability to be empathetic.

- **Difficult patient behavior**: Some patients may be reticent, aggressive or depressed, making interaction more complex.

To overcome these obstacles, it is essential that the caregiver takes care of himself, recognizes his limits and seeks support from his colleagues or hierarchy if necessary.

Strategies for developing empathy and patience

1. **Ongoing training**
   Participate in workshops and training courses on empathic communication, stress management and relaxation techniques.

2. **Self-reflection**
   Take the time to reflect on your own reactions, identify situations that give rise to impatience or irritation, and develop strategies for dealing with them.

3. **Mindfulness practice**
   Meditation and mindfulness exercises can help you stay present, manage your emotions and improve your listening skills.

4. **Colleague support**
   Sharing experiences and challenges with the team provides advice, fresh perspectives and moral support.

Positive impact on quality of care

By integrating empathy and patience into daily practice, the caregiver contributes to :

- **Better adherence to care**: Patients are more likely to follow recommendations and actively participate in their rehabilitation.

- **Reduced complications**: A patient who feels understood and supported is less stressed, which can have a positive impact on his or her overall health.

- **Improved patient experience**: Feeling respected and valued enhances patients' psychological well-being and satisfaction with the care they receive.

Concrete examples from a care situation

- **Accompanying the patient on journeys**
  If a patient has difficulty getting around, the caregiver shows patience by gently guiding them, explaining each step, without rushing them. Empathy is shown by recognizing the stress this situation can cause the patient.

- **Learning new technologies**
  When introducing an assistive device, the caregiver calmly explains how it works, repeats instructions if necessary, and encourages the patient to ask questions. He or she understands that learning can be intimidating, and offers appropriate support.

- **Dealing with strong emotions**
  If the patient expresses anger or sadness, the caregiver

listens without judgment, validates feelings ("I understand how difficult this can be for you") and suggests solutions or additional support.

Ethics and deontology

Ethics and deontology play a central role in the daily practice of care for blind people. These principles guide professional actions, ensure respect for the rights and dignity of patients, and foster a relationship of trust essential to quality care. Understanding and integrating these notions is essential to meeting the moral demands of the profession, and to navigating the complex situations that may arise with integrity.

The foundations of professional ethics

Ethics in healthcare are based on fundamental principles that guide decision-making and behavior:

1. **Respect for autonomy**: Recognizing patients' right to make decisions about their own health and well-being. This means providing clear information, respecting their choices and supporting their independence.

2. **Beneficence**: Acting in the patient's best interests, aiming to promote well-being and prevent harm.

3. **Non-maleficence**: Avoid causing harm to the patient, whether by action or omission.

4. **Justice**: Treating every patient fairly, without discrimination, and ensuring an equitable distribution of resources and care.

5. **Confidentiality**: Respecting patient privacy by protecting personal and medical information.

Applying ethical principles in daily practice

1. **Respect for patient dignity and autonomy**

    - **Informed consent**: Before any intervention, the caregiver must ensure that the patient understands the procedures to be carried out and consents freely to them. This requires appropriate communication to compensate for vision loss.

    - **Promoting autonomy**: Encouraging patients to actively participate in their own care, to make decisions about their treatment, and to develop their skills for greater independence.

    - **Avoid overprotection**: Although the intention is to protect the patient, excessive assistance can hinder his or her autonomy and self-confidence.

2. **Confidentiality and privacy**

    - **Protecting information**: Only divulge patient medical information to the professionals concerned and with the patient's consent.

    - **Discretion in discussion**: Avoid discussing patients' cases in public places or with people not involved in their care.

    - **Respect for privacy**: During treatment, take care to preserve the patient's privacy, for example by closing the door or covering untreated parts of the body.

3. **Beneficence and non-maleficence**

    - **Quality care**: Providing care based on best practices, keeping abreast of medical and technological advances.

    - **Risk prevention**: Identify and minimize potential hazards to the patient, such as obstacles in the environment or medication errors.

    - **Error management**: In the event of an error or incident, inform the patient honestly, take the necessary corrective action and prevent recurrences.

4. **Fairness and equity**

    - **Equal treatment**: Offering the same level of care and attention to all patients, regardless of their origin, socio-economic status, religion or any other factor.

    - **Access to resources**: Inform patients about available services and assistance, and help them access them if necessary.

    - **Anti-discrimination**: Be vigilant in the face of discriminatory attitudes or practices, and denounce them if necessary.

Professional ethics

Ethics are the rules and duties that govern a profession. For caregivers, this includes :

1. **Compliance with the Code of Ethics**

    - **Professional competence**: Keep skills up to date through ongoing training and apply knowledge diligently.

    - **Integrity**: Act with honesty, avoid conflicts of interest, and do not abuse your position.

    - **Responsibility**: Taking responsibility for one's actions, respecting protocols and procedures, and collaborating with the care team.

2. **Business relations**

    - **Teamwork**: Collaborate with other healthcare professionals in a spirit of mutual respect, open communication and complementarity.

    - **Respect for hierarchies and competencies**: Recognize the limits of your role, refer to the appropriate professionals if necessary, and follow medical directives.

    - **Conflict management**: deal with disagreements constructively, emphasizing dialogue and the search for solutions.

3. **Commitment to the patient**

    - **Patient advocacy**: Act as the patient's advocate, ensuring that his or her needs are met, and representing him or her when necessary with other professionals.

    - **Empathy and respect**: Treat patients with courtesy, understanding and non-judgment.

- **Honest communication**: Provide truthful information, adapted to the patient's understanding, and avoid false promises.

Complex ethical situations

In practice, the caregiver may be faced with ethical dilemmas, such as:

1. **Refusal of care**
   If a blind patient refuses treatment or assistance, the caregiver must respect his or her choice, while ensuring that he or she is fully informed of the consequences. This may require discussion with the medical team, or the involvement of a mediator.

2. **Confidentiality in the face of risk**
   If the patient discloses information suggesting danger to him/herself or others (e.g. suicidal thoughts), the caregiver must assess the need to break confidentiality to protect the patient, following established protocols.

3. **Family pressures**
   The family's views on care may differ from those of the patient. The caregiver must support the patient's autonomy, facilitate communication between the parties and, if necessary, call on mediation services.

Ethics training and support

To navigate these situations effectively, it is important that the caregiver :

- **Receive ethics training**: Understand ethical principles, relevant laws and regulations, and develop ethical decision-making skills.

- **Participate in ethical discussions**: Team meetings, focus groups or ethics committees can provide forums for discussing complex cases and sharing perspectives.
- **Access resources**: Guides, codes of ethics and institutional protocols can serve as references to guide actions.

Applicable laws and regulations

Ethical practice is supported by a legal framework that protects the rights of patients and defines the obligations of professionals:

- **Public Health Code**: governs the healthcare professions, including provisions on professional secrecy, informed consent and patients' rights.
- **The law of March 4, 2002 on patients' rights and the quality of the healthcare system**: reinforces patients' right to information, consent and participation in decisions concerning them.
- **Patient rights charters**: Institutional documents setting out the fundamental principles to be respected in patient care.

The caregiver's role in promoting ethics

The caregiver is not only a care provider, but also a key player in promoting ethical practice:

- **Ensure patient rights are respected**: Be alert to situations where the patient's rights could be compromised and intervene or alert if necessary.

- **Model of ethical behavior**: By adopting exemplary conduct, the caregiver positively influences colleagues and contributes to a culture of respect and integrity.
- **Patient education**: informing patients of their rights, encouraging them to express their wishes and actively participate in their care.

Interprofessional collaboration

Caring for blind people is a complex task, requiring the involvement of multiple health and social care professionals. The caregiver, as an essential member of the care team, plays a pivotal role in this inter-professional collaboration. Understanding the importance of this cooperation, and knowing how to actively participate in it, is crucial to ensuring comprehensive, effective and patient-centered care.

The importance of interprofessional collaboration

Blindness affects not only vision, but also mobility, communication, mental health, social integration and the patient's overall quality of life. No single professional can meet all these needs. Interprofessional collaboration brings together the complementary skills of different specialists to offer a holistic approach to care.

This collaboration promotes :

- **Better coordination of care**: It avoids redundancies and oversights, and ensures continuity of care between the various parties involved.
- **Shared decision-making**: Varied perspectives enrich the development of personalized care plans.
- **Improved patient outcomes**: A collaborative approach responds more effectively to complex patient needs.

- **Professional support**: Teamwork enables us to share responsibilities, exchange knowledge and support each other in the face of professional challenges.

Key players in interprofessional collaboration

1. **Ophthalmologists**
   Specialists in eye diseases, they are responsible for the diagnosis, medical and surgical treatment of eye pathologies. They assess the extent of visual impairment, monitor disease progression and determine the necessary interventions.

2. **Nurses**
   They provide daily medical care, administer prescribed treatments, monitor clinical signs and play an educational role with the patient. Their close collaboration with the caregiver is essential to ensure continuity of care.

3. **Orthoptists**
   Specialized in visual rehabilitation, they help patients optimize their residual vision, teaching techniques to improve eye movement coordination and adaptation to visual aids.

4. **Occupational therapists**
   They assess the patient's functional abilities and propose adaptations to the environment to facilitate activities of daily living. They teach methods to compensate for vision loss and promote autonomy.

5. **Psychologists and psychiatrists**
   They offer psychological support to help patients cope with the emotional impact of blindness, such as depression, anxiety or adapting to lifestyle changes.

6. **Social workers**
    Inform patients about their rights, available financial assistance, community resources and support programs. They facilitate access to social services and coordinate the necessary interventions.

7. **Rehabilitation professionals**
    These include orientation and mobility specialists, who teach patients how to move around safely, using a white cane or other assistive devices.

8. **Specialized educators**
    They work with patients, especially children, to develop educational, social and communication skills adapted to their condition.

9. **Family and caregivers**
    Although they are not healthcare professionals, their involvement is crucial. They provide day-to-day support, participate in decision-making and collaborate with professionals to ensure the patient's well-being.

The caregiver's role in interprofessional collaboration

The caregiver occupies a unique position, often being the professional closest to the patient in day-to-day care. Their responsibilities in interprofessional collaboration include :

- **Observation and transmission of information**
  Through regular contact with the patient, the caregiver is well placed to observe changes in health status, reactions to treatment and emerging needs. They must communicate these observations effectively to other team members, so that care can be adjusted accordingly.

- **Participation in coordination meetings**
  By attending team meetings, caregivers can share their perspectives, contribute to care planning and keep abreast of what other professionals are doing.

- **Implementing care plans**
  He applies the recommendations of other professionals, such as the exercises prescribed by the occupational therapist or the communication techniques suggested by the psychologist.

- **Patient education and support**
  The caregiver reinforces the information provided by other professionals, helps the patient understand the objectives of the various interventions and encourages his or her active participation.

- **Facilitating communication**
  It can act as a liaison between the patient and the team, ensuring that the patient's concerns are heard and that information is conveyed clearly and appropriately.

Skills required for effective collaboration

1. **Clear, open communication**
   Use professional, precise and respectful language. Ensure messages are clearly understood and regularly check mutual understanding.

2. **Respect and recognition of each other's skills**
   Valuing the contributions of other professionals, understanding the roles and responsibilities of each, and avoiding judgments or territorial conflicts.

3. **Flexibility and adaptability** Be ready to adjust actions in response to new information or changes in the care plan. Accept constructive feedback and be open to continuous learning.

4. **Confidentiality and ethics**
   Share relevant information while respecting the rules of confidentiality and the ethical principles of the profession.

5. **Team spirit**
   Foster a climate of collaboration, support colleagues and contribute to a positive team dynamic.

Challenges of interprofessional collaboration

- **Communication barriers**
  Differences in terminology, professional culture and communication methods can lead to misunderstandings. It's important to clarify messages and develop a common language.

- **Different priorities or perspectives**
  Professionals may have different approaches based on their training or experience. Open discussion and mutual respect are essential to reconcile these differences.

- **Organizational constraints**
  Busy schedules, complex healthcare systems or lack of resources can complicate collaboration. Planning and coordination are needed to overcome these obstacles.

Strategies for strengthening collaboration

1. **Interprofessional training**
   Participate in training courses or workshops that bring together different professionals to learn together and understand each other's roles.

2. **Use of shared communication tools**
   Adopt shared electronic patient records, secure communication platforms or standardized protocols to facilitate information exchange.

3. **Development of common protocols** Establish integrated care plans and procedures that reflect the contributions of each professional and ensure a consistent approach.

4. **Encouraging a collaborative culture**
   Organizations can promote collaborative values, recognize and reward team efforts, and support initiatives that foster interprofessional working.

Positive impact on the patient

Effective interprofessional collaboration means :

- **Patient-centred care**
  By combining their expertise, professionals can offer personalized care that meets the patient's specific needs.

- **Greater patient satisfaction**
  Patients benefit from coherent care, a better understanding of their care pathway and the support of a united team.

- **Improved health outcomes**
  Coordinated interventions reduce the risk of errors, improve treatment efficiency and promote optimal recovery.

Chapter 3

Appropriate communication techniques

Effective verbal communication

Verbal communication is central to the relationship between the caregiver and the blind patient. It is the principal means by which information is conveyed, care explained, and emotional support offered. Effective verbal communication goes far beyond the simple transmission of messages; it involves attentive listening, clear expression and constant adaptation to the patient's specific needs. In the absence of visual cues, every word and every intonation takes on added importance, making mastery of this skill essential to quality care.

The importance of verbal communication for blind patients

Loss of vision deprives the patient of much of the environmental and social information usually perceived through visual signals. Facial expressions, gestures and body language are all elements of non-verbal communication that are no longer accessible. The blind patient therefore relies more on hearing to understand his environment and interact with others. Caregivers must be aware of this and adapt their communication accordingly, emphasizing clarity, precision and human warmth in their verbal exchanges.

Fundamentals of effective verbal communication

1. **Introduce yourself clearly and announce your presence** At every meeting, it's essential to introduce yourself or remind people who you are. For example: "Hello, Mr. Dupont, I'm Claire, your caregiver. I've just come into your room. This helps patients understand who is talking to them and establishes a relationship of trust.

2. **Explain each action before carrying it out**
Before taking any action, tell the patient what you're going to do, why and how. For example: "I'm now going to help you stand up. I'm going to place my hand under

your right arm to support you." This avoids unpleasant surprises and allows the patient to prepare mentally and physically.

3. **Use clear, precise language** Avoid unexplained technical terms or ambiguous expressions. Use simple, direct sentences, making sure you articulate correctly. For example: "Your medication is on the table in front of you, about thirty centimetres away.

4. **Adapt tone and rhythm of voice**
   Speak in a soft, calm, steady voice. Avoid shouting or speaking too quickly. Your tone of voice should reflect kindness and respect.

5. **Avoid purely visual expressions**
   Replace expressions like "Look here" or "You see" with "Listen", "I'll explain" or "Do you understand". This makes communication more appropriate and respectful of the patient's situation.

6. **Giving temporal and spatial cues**
   Inform the patient of temporal elements (time of day, course of the day) and spatial elements (room layout, location of objects). For example: "It's 8 a.m., breakfast will be served in 30 minutes.

7. **Check patient comprehension**
   Make sure the patient has grasped the information by asking open-ended questions. For example, "Do you have any questions about what I've just explained?" or "Would you like me to repeat any information?"

8. **Encouraging patient expression**
   Invite patients to share their feelings, concerns or needs. Listen carefully to responses without interrupting, and respond with empathy.

Specific techniques to improve communication

- **Using the patient's name**
  Calling the patient by name makes it easier to personalize the relationship and capture his or her attention. It also reinforces the bond of trust.

- **Taking audible non-verbal language into account**
  Sighs, hesitations and the tone of a patient's voice can reveal his or her emotions or needs. Being attentive to these signals enables you to adapt your response appropriately.

- **Avoid noise distractions**
  Reduce ambient noise as much as possible to facilitate patient concentration and understanding. Turn off the TV or radio if necessary.

- **Adapting distance and position**
  Face the patient, at a comfortable conversational distance. Even if eye contact is not possible, this position facilitates interaction.

Managing complex or delicate situations

- **Approach sensitive subjects with tact**
  When it comes to difficult discussions (bad news, treatment changes), choose an appropriate moment and adopt an empathetic approach.

- **Responding to the patient's emotions**
  If the patient expresses anger, sadness or anxiety, acknowledge these emotions and offer support. For example: "I understand that you feel worried about this. Talk to me about what's bothering you."

- **Maintain a professional attitude**
  Remain calm and patient, even in the face of frustration

or disagreement. Avoid taking patient reactions personally.

Promoting patient autonomy through communication

- **Give clear instructions for daily activities**
  Explain the steps involved in tasks that the patient can perform on his or her own, providing verbal guidance. For example: "To get dressed, your clothes are laid out on the bed, with the pants on the left and the sweater on the right."

- **Encouraging decision-making**
  Offer patients choices and respect their preferences. For example: "Would you prefer to shower now or after breakfast?

- **Providing educational information**
  Inform patients about their condition, treatments and rehabilitation exercises, adapting the level of detail to their understanding.

Using technology to support communication

- **Text-to-speech devices and screen readers**
  These tools enable patients to access written information, read documents or surf the Internet.

- **Adapted mobile applications**
  There are applications designed to help blind people with various tasks, such as text recognition, image description or localization.

- **Device training**
  The caregiver can help the patient become familiar with these technologies, by providing clear instructions and answering questions.

Teamwork for coherent communication

- **Coordination with colleagues**
  Share important information about patient preferences and needs with the care team to ensure a consistent approach.

- **Exchange best practices**
  Discuss effective communication techniques and challenges encountered to continuously improve the quality of interactions.

- **Participate in group training**
  Communication workshops can strengthen team skills and promote a better understanding of blindness-related issues.

Respecting confidentiality and ethics

- **Protecting personal information**
  Patient information must not be disclosed to unauthorized third parties. Discussions concerning the patient should take place in private areas.

- **Obtaining consent**
  Before sharing information with other professionals or family members, make sure the patient agrees.

- **Adopt a respectful attitude** Avoid judgments, stereotypes or prejudices. Treat patients with dignity and consideration.

Body language and therapeutic touch

In the care of blind people, body language and therapeutic touch are of particular importance. Although blind patients cannot perceive visual signals such as facial expressions or gestures, body language remains an essential means of communication, mainly through tone of voice, posture and touch. Understanding and mastering these elements enables the caregiver to establish a relationship of trust, convey information effectively and provide appropriate emotional support.

The role of body language in communication with blind patients

1. **Vocal expression as an extension of body language**

    - **Intonation and voice modulation**: The tone, rhythm and volume of the voice convey emotions and intentions. A calm, warm voice can reassure the patient, while a brusque or monotonous tone can create anxiety or confusion.

    - **Smile in the voice**: Even if the patient can't see a smile, it can be heard in the voice. Adopting a positive attitude is reflected in the way you speak and can put the patient at ease.

2. **Posture and physical presence**

    - **Body orientation**: Positioning yourself in front of the patient when speaking, even if they can't see you, makes it easier to project your voice and shows respect.

    - **Interpersonal distance**: Maintaining an appropriate distance, neither too close nor too far, contributes to a comfortable exchange. Excessive proximity can be intrusive, while too great a distance can give the impression of detachment.

3. **Body movements and noises**

    ○ **Avoid sudden movements**: Sudden noises or rapid movements can startle the patient. It's important to move calmly and signal your actions.

    ○ **Notifying your presence**: Letting the patient know when you are entering or leaving the room avoids misunderstandings and feelings of abandonment.

Touch as a means of communication and care

Touch is a particularly well-developed sense for blind people, and a powerful channel of communication. It can convey security, comfort and empathy. However, it must be used with discernment and respect for individual preferences.

1. **Principles of therapeutic touch**

    ○ **Consent**: Always ask permission before touching the patient. For example, "May I put my hand on your shoulder to guide you?"

    ○ **Respect for sensitive areas**: Avoid touching areas of the body that could be perceived as intrusive or inappropriate, such as the face, chest or intimate areas, unless necessary for care and with the patient's explicit consent.

    ○ **Appropriate pressure and duration**: A light, brief touch is generally preferable. Excessive pressure or prolonged contact can be uncomfortable.

2. Applications of touch in care

- **Physical guidance**: When it's necessary to help the patient move around, suggest that he or she holds the caregiver's arm, rather than pushing or pulling. This gives the patient control over movement and reinforces his or her autonomy.

- **Emotional support**: A gentle touch, such as a hand on the forearm, can offer comfort during difficult times. It's important to ensure that the patient is receptive to this kind of contact.

- **Specific therapeutic techniques**: In certain situations, light massage or tactile exercises can be used to relieve pain, reduce anxiety or improve blood circulation. Proper training is required to apply these techniques correctly.

3. Tactile communication

- **Use of Braille**: Encouraging patients to learn Braille enables them to read and write independently, enhancing their communication and access to information.

- **Tactile cues in the environment**: Installing tactile cues, such as different textures on door handles or light switches, helps patients to orientate themselves and interact with their environment independently.

Cultural and personal considerations

Perceptions of touch vary according to culture, religion and individual experience. What is acceptable to one person may not be to another.

- **Cultural sensitivity**: Be aware of the patient's cultural norms regarding physical contact. For example, in some cultures, contact between people of the opposite sex may be restricted.

- **Personal preferences**: Every patient has his or her own limits when it comes to touch. It's essential to discuss with them what makes them feel comfortable, and to respect their wishes.

Caregiver training and skills

To use body language and therapeutic touch effectively, the caregiver must develop certain skills:

1. **Self-awareness**

    - **Become aware of your own body language**: Even if the patient can't see it, adopting an open, relaxed posture has a positive influence on your tone of voice and general attitude.

    - **Managing emotions**: Feelings of stress or impatience can be reflected in your voice or gestures. Learning to manage your emotions helps maintain calm communication.

2. **Specific training**

    - **Therapeutic touch techniques**: Training to master appropriate methods of touch in a healthcare context.

    - **Adapted non-verbal communication**: Attend workshops or training courses on communicating with blind people to hone your skills.

3. **Empathy and active listening**

    ○ **Paying attention to the patient's reactions**: Even without eye contact, patients express their feelings through their tone of voice, breathing and posture. Paying attention to these cues enables you to adjust your approach.

    ○ **Encourage feedback**: Invite patients to express their preferences or discomforts regarding touch or communication in general.

Professional ethics and limits

The use of touch must always respect ethical and professional limits:

- **Maintaining a professional relationship**: Touch must serve the patient's well-being and be part of the care process.

- **Privacy**: Protect patient privacy by ensuring that procedures involving physical contact take place in an appropriate environment.

- **Ongoing consent**: Consent to touch is not acquired once and for all. It is important to check regularly that the patient is still comfortable with physical contact.

Practical examples

1. **Mobility assistance**
   When the patient needs to move around, suggest: "May I offer you my arm to guide you to the dining room?" With the patient holding the arm, walk slightly forward, describing obstacles or changes in direction.

2. **Personal care**
   During personal care, explain each step: "Now I'll help

you wash your face. If you prefer to do it yourself, I can give you the washcloth."

3. **Emotional support**

    If the patient expresses distress, ask: "Would you like me to stay with you?" If appropriate, a gentle touch on the shoulder can provide comfort.

Use of assistive technologies

The advent of assistive technologies has revolutionized the care of blind people, offering innovative solutions to improve their autonomy, communication and social integration. These tools, which encompass a wide range of hardware and software devices, compensate for vision loss by exploiting other senses, notably hearing and touch. For the caregiver, mastery of these technologies is essential in order to effectively support the patient in their use and maximize the benefits they can bring to their quality of life.

The main assistive technologies for blind people

1. **Screen-reading and text-to-speech devices**

    Screen-reading software is a computer program that interprets the content displayed on a computer or smartphone screen and renders it in speech or Braille via a Braille display. They enable blind people to access digital information, browse the Internet, manage their e-mail and use various applications.

    ○ **JAWS (Job Access With Speech)**: One of the most widely used screen-reading programs for Windows computers. It offers high-quality text-to-speech and advanced features for efficient navigation.

- **NVDA (NonVisual Desktop Access)**: A free, open-source alternative to JAWS, compatible with Windows, offering speech synthesis and support for Braille displays.

- **VoiceOver**: Integrated into Apple devices (macOS, iOS), it enables smooth voice navigation on Mac computers, iPhones and iPads.

- **TalkBack**: The screen reader for Android devices, offering voice synthesis and adapted gesture commands.

2. **Braille displays and keyboards**
Braille displays are devices that transform digital text into tactile Braille characters, enabling users to read information with their fingers. They are often used in conjunction with screen readers.

    - **Portable Braille displays**: Small in size, they connect to smartphones or computers, making it easy to read on the move.

    - **Braille notepad**: Combination of a Braille display and a Braille keyboard, enabling you to take notes, read documents and manage tasks independently.

3. **Specific mobile applications**
Smartphones have become indispensable tools, thanks to a host of applications designed to help blind people.

    - **Be My Eyes**: Connects blind people with sighted volunteers via a live video connection for help with everyday tasks.

    - **Seeing AI**: Developed by Microsoft, this application uses artificial intelligence to describe objects, texts, people and scenes captured by the smartphone's camera.

- **Lookout**: A similar application for Android, using AI to recognize objects and text.

- **Voice Dream Reader**: A document and audiobook reader with advanced customization options.

4. **Navigation and mobility technologies**

    - **Adapted GPS**: Applications such as **BlindSquare** or **GoodMaps** provide precise navigation information, adapted to the needs of blind people, describing the environment and indicating nearby points of interest.

    - **Audible beacons**: Installed in certain public spaces, they emit sound signals or voice messages to aid orientation.

    - **Electronic cane**: Equipped with ultrasonic or laser sensors, it detects obstacles at a distance and alerts the user with vibrations or sound signals.

5. **Assistive reading and writing devices**

    - **Electronic magnifiers**: Portable devices that magnify and display text on a screen with high-contrast options.

    - **Optical character recognition (OCR) systems**: convert printed documents into digital text that can be read by voice synthesis or Braille. For example, the **OrCam MyEye**, a small camera attached to glasses that reads text aloud in real time.

6. **Home automation assistance technologies**

    - **Voice assistants**: devices such as **Amazon Echo** (Alexa), **Google Home** or **Apple HomePod allow** home appliances to be controlled by voice, making it easier to access information, manage household chores and enjoy entertainment.

    - **Connected objects**: Thermostats, lighting, locks and other devices compatible with voice commands, improving independence at home.

The role of the caregiver in the use of assistive technologies

1. **Patient needs assessment**

    - **Customized analysis**: Understanding the patient's specific needs, capabilities and preferences to select the most appropriate technologies.

    - **Collaboration with specialists**: Work with occupational therapists, orthoptists or specialized technicians for in-depth assessment.

2. **Training and support**

    - **Introduction to technologies**: Explain how devices work, demonstrate their use and assist patients with their first manipulations.

    - **Adapted pedagogy**: Adapt the pace and method of learning to the patient's skills, being patient and encouraging.

    - **Accessible documentation**: Provide user guides in Braille, large print or audio format.

3. **Technical assistance**

    - **Device configuration**: Helping to install, update and customize settings to meet patient needs.

    - **Problem solving**: Be able to diagnose common problems and propose solutions or call on technical support if necessary.

4. **Promoting autonomy**

    - **Encouraging daily use**: Integrating technologies into patients' routines to reinforce their autonomy and self-confidence.

    - **Ongoing support**: Remain available to answer questions, adjust configurations or introduce new features as the patient becomes familiar with the tools.

5. **Raising awareness of new technologies**

    - **Technology watch**: keep abreast of innovations and updates in the field of assistive technologies.

    - **Patient information**: Present new solutions that could improve the patient's quality of life, by assessing their relevance together.

Issues and challenges related to the use of assistive technologies

1. **Financial accessibility**

    - **Cost of devices**: Some equipment can be expensive, limiting accessibility.

- **Financial assistance**: Inform the patient about the possibilities of coverage, subsidies or assistance programs available.

2. **Technological barriers**

    - **Complexity of tools**: Some patients may be reluctant or find it difficult to use advanced technologies.

    - **Insufficient training** : Lack of training can lead to under-utilization or abandonment of devices.

3. **Maintenance and updates**

    - **Obsolescence**: Technologies evolve rapidly, requiring regular updates.

    - **Technical support**: Ensure access to reliable technical support to resolve any problems.

4. **Security and confidentiality**

    - **Data protection**: Make patients aware of the risks associated with confidentiality, particularly with connected devices.

    - **Best practices**: Encourage the use of secure passwords, and caution when sharing personal information.

The benefits of assistive technologies for blind patients

- **Greater autonomy**: technologies enable people to carry out everyday tasks without assistance, reinforcing their independence.

- **Access to information**: Facilitating access to education, culture, news and leisure.

- **Enhanced communication**: Keep in touch with loved ones, participate in social networks and online communities.

- **Social integration**: more active participation in community, professional and social life.

- **Improved quality of life**: Reduced feelings of isolation, increased self-confidence and general well-being.

Chapter 4

Assistance with activities of daily living

Mobility and orientation

- **Guiding techniques**

Mobility is a fundamental aspect of independence for blind people. As a caregiver, it is essential to master guiding techniques in order to accompany patients safely and respectfully. Effective guidance is based on clear communication, an understanding of the patient's individual needs and the application of methods adapted to different situations.

General guidance principles

1. **Offering assistance with respect**
   Before you start guiding a blind person, it's important to offer your help in a courteous, non-intrusive way. Say, for example, "Hello, can I help you get around? Respect their response, whether positive or negative, and never impose your assistance.

2. **Appropriate guiding position**
   Once you've accepted the aid, position yourself slightly in front of the patient, on the side he/she prefers. Offer him your arm, bending it at right angles, so that he can hold your elbow or forearm. This position enables the patient to feel your movements and anticipate changes in direction or rhythm.

3. **Clear verbal communication**
   Inform the patient of each stage of the route: obstacles, changes of direction, climbs, descents, etc. Use precise language and avoid ambiguous terms. For example, instead of saying "Be careful", say "There's a step up ahead".

4. **Adapting your walking pace**
Adapt your pace to that of the patient. Walk at a steady pace and avoid sudden movements. If you need to slow down or speed up, let the patient know in advance.

5. **Respecting autonomy**
Encourage patients to use their skills and technical aids, such as a white cane or guide dog, to complement your guidance. Respect the patient's mobility preferences.

Specific guiding techniques

1. **Passing through doors**
   - **Door approach**: Inform the patient when arriving at a door and specify whether it opens inwards or outwards, and which side the handle is on.
   - **Passing through** : Go through the door first, holding it open with your hand opposite the patient. The patient will continue to hold your arm and will be able to feel the movement.
   - **Transition**: Once through the door, return to your initial guiding position.

2. **Stairs and steps**
   - **Announcement**: Clearly state whether you're going up or down stairs, and mention the approximate number of steps if possible.
   - **Positioning**: Before the staircase, stop briefly to allow the patient to prepare. Position yourself slightly forward.
   - **Handrail**: If a handrail is available, guide the patient's hand towards it.
   - **Pace**: Go up or down at a steady pace, informing the patient of the last step.

3. **Passage through narrow spaces**

    - **Warning**: Warn the patient that the passageway is narrowing.
    - **Single-file position**: Place your arm behind your back; the patient moves his hand to your wrist to position himself behind you.
    - **Resuming normal position**: Once the space has been cleared, signal to the patient that he/she can return to the original position.

4. **Changes of direction**

    - **Anticipation**: Inform the patient a few steps before the change of direction.
    - **Hint**: Use clear terms like "We're going to turn left" or "We're making a U-turn".
    - **Coordinated movement**: Turn gently, allowing the patient to follow your movement naturally.

5. **Seating assistance**

    - **Seat location**: Inform the patient of the presence of a chair or armchair, describing its position and orientation.
    - **Tactile guidance**: Place the patient's hand on the seat back or armrest.
    - **Stability**: Make sure the seat is stable before the patient sits down.

6. **Crossing the street**

    - **Safety**: Check that the lane is clear and inform the patient when it's time to cross.
    - **Additional information**: Mention the presence of traffic lights, crosswalks or any construction work.

- **Adapted pace**: Cross at a comfortable pace, keeping an eye out for unexpected obstacles.

7. **Use of public transport**

    - **Getting into the vehicle**: Indicate the number of steps or the height of the step. Guide the patient to an available grab bar or seat.
    - **During the journey**: Inform him of upcoming stops and estimated journey times.
    - **Getting off the vehicle**: Help the patient prepare for the descent by announcing the approach of the stop.

Practical tips for efficient guidance

- **Constant communication**: Stay in dialogue with the patient, encouraging them to ask questions or express their needs.
- **Adaptability**: Every person is different. Adapt your techniques to the patient's preferences and abilities.
- **Ongoing training**: Keep abreast of best practice in guiding, and attend specialist training courses where possible.
- **Empathy and respect**: Be patient and understanding. Avoid making the patient feel like a burden.

Mistakes to avoid

- **Not anticipating obstacles**: It's crucial to inform the patient of obstacles in advance to avoid accidents.
- **Imposing help**: Respect refusal to help. Never force a person to accept your guidance.
- **Lack of communication**: Don't assume the patient knows what's going on. A lack of information can generate anxiety.

Use of mobility aids

- **White cane**: If the patient uses a cane, walk beside him, adapting your pace. The cane enables him to detect obstacles on the ground.
- **Guide dog**: When the patient is accompanied by a guide dog, walk on the opposite side to the dog. Do not distract the dog while it is working.
- **Electronic devices**: Some patients use mobile applications or navigation devices. Be open to integrating these tools into your support.

The importance of practice

Mastery of guiding techniques comes with experience. Don't hesitate to :

- **Simulate situations**: Train with colleagues to perfect your gestures and communication skills.
- **Ask for feedback**: Solicit patients' opinions on the way you guide to help you improve.
- **Watching experienced professionals**: learn techniques and tips from those trained in guiding.

- **Travel safety**

Mobility is a fundamental element in the autonomy and quality of life of blind people. Being able to move around safely not only enables them to carry out daily activities, but also to participate fully in social, professional and cultural life. As a caregiver, you play a crucial role in accompanying blind patients to ensure their safety when moving around. This requires a thorough understanding of potential risks, a mastery of appropriate techniques and an awareness of the specific needs of each individual.

Understanding the challenges of safety on the move

Blind people face many challenges when getting around. Lack of vision exposes them to physical obstacles, environmental hazards and unexpected situations that can lead to injury or accidents. What's more, the lack of visual cues can lead to anxiety or confusion, affecting their self-confidence and willingness to move around independently.

Ensuring safe travel therefore involves :

- **Identify and minimize risks**: Recognize potential hazards in the environment and take steps to eliminate or mitigate them.
- **Provide appropriate support**: Use appropriate guidance techniques and offer personalized support based on the patient's abilities and preferences.
- **Encouraging autonomy**: helping patients to develop the skills needed to move around safely on their own, using technical aids or compensatory strategies.
- **Creating a safe environment**: Adapt living and working spaces so that they are accessible and free of obstacles.

Risk assessment and travel planning

Before any move, it is important to carry out a risk assessment specific to the environment and the patient:

1. **Environmental analysis**

    - **Identifying obstacles**: Locate furniture, objects or structures that could impede passage, such as carpets, electrical cables, unmarked steps or misaligned doors.
    - **Assessment of floor conditions**: Check for slippery, uneven or cluttered surfaces that could lead to falls.

- **Lighting control**: Although the patient is blind, adequate lighting can help caregivers spot hazards and facilitate communication.

2. **Knowledge of the patient's abilities**

    - **Mobility and balance**: Assess the patient's stability, physical strength and ability to move around with or without assistance.
    - **Use of technical aids**: Determine whether the patient uses a white cane, a guide dog or electronic devices, and whether he or she has mastered their use.
    - **Emotional state**: Take into account any anxiety, fatigue or stress that could affect the safety of the trip.

3. **Route planning**

    - **Choice of route**: Choose the most direct, well-known paths with no major obstacles.
    - **Preparing the patient**: Inform the patient of the planned route, points of interest and any changes to their routine.
    - **Plan breaks**: If the journey is long, plan rest periods to avoid fatigue.

Techniques for ensuring safety on the move

1. **Appropriate use of mobility aids**

    - **White cane**: The cane is an essential tool for detecting obstacles on the ground. Make sure the patient is trained to use it, and encourage its systematic use.
    - **Guide dog**: If the patient has a guide dog, follow the specific instructions for its use. Do not distract the dog during its work, and inform the

patient of anything that could affect it (presence of other animals, unusual obstacles).
- **Electronic devices**: Technologies such as voice-activated GPS applications can help with navigation. Make sure the patient knows how to use them and that they are properly configured.

2. Environmental planning

- **Space organization**: Keep furniture in a constant arrangement so that patients can easily find their way around. Avoid leaving objects lying around on the floor.
- **Tactile and auditory signage**: Install tactile cues, such as rumble strips on steps or floor markings. Use audible signals to indicate certain locations (door chimes, beepers on crosswalks).
- **Lighting**: Even if the patient is blind, good lighting can help the sighted people accompanying him/her, and improve contrast perception for visually impaired patients.

3. Training in independent mobility techniques

- **Orientation and mobility**: Work with specialized professionals to teach patients orientation techniques based on sounds, smells, ground textures or thermal sensations.
- **Counting strategies**: Learn to count steps or course elements (such as gates or intersections) to find your bearings.
- **Obstacle management**: Teach how to approach stairs, sidewalks, ramps and other structural elements safely.

4. **Effective communication**

    - **Precise descriptions**: Inform the patient in real time about the characteristics of the environment, upcoming obstacles and actions to be taken.
    - **Clear language**: Use precise terms, avoid ambiguity. For example, say "There are three steps to climb" rather than "Watch out for the steps".
    - **Checking comprehension**: Make sure the patient has understood the information provided, and encourage questions.

Accident prevention and emergency management

1. **Anticipating hazards**

    - **Constant vigilance**: Staying alert to the environment to detect potential hazards before they become obstacles for the patient.
    - **Adapting to change**: Be prepared to modify the route in the event of unforeseen circumstances, such as construction work, crowds or adverse weather conditions.

2. **First aid training**

    - **Basic skills**: Master first-aid techniques to react quickly in the event of a fall, injury or discomfort.
    - **Emergency plan**: Know the procedures to follow in the event of an emergency, the numbers to call and the information to provide.

3. **Emotional support**

    - **Stress management**: Help patients remain calm in unexpected situations. Use a reassuring tone and give clear instructions.
    - **Encouragement**: boost patients' confidence by recognizing their skills and efforts.

Collaboration with the interdisciplinary team

1. **Networking**

    - **Coordination with professionals**: Collaborate with occupational therapists, locomotion instructors, psychologists and other professionals to develop safe mobility plans.
    - **Information sharing**: Communicate observations and concerns about patient safety to team members for consistent management.

2. **Involving family and friends**

    - **Awareness**: Inform relatives about guidance techniques and safety measures, so that they can support the patient's movements.
    - **Emotional support**: Encourage the family to participate in the rehabilitation process and support the patient's autonomy.

Knowledge updating and continuing education

1. **Updating skills**

    - **Specialized training** : Participate in workshops or training courses on new assistance technologies, mobility techniques and innovative approaches to safety.

- **Professional watch**: Keep abreast of research and publications in the field of blindness and mobility.

2. **Reflections on practice**

    - **Self-assessment**: Regularly analyze practices to identify strengths and areas for improvement.
    - **Patient feedback**: Solicit the patient's opinion on the support provided and take their suggestions into account to improve safety and comfort.

Promoting autonomy and self-confidence

1. **Encouraging independence**

    - **Gradual progression**: Helping patients to gradually acquire the skills needed to move around independently in familiar and then unfamiliar environments.
    - **Setting realistic goals**: Establish mobility goals with the patient that are adapted to his or her abilities and aspirations.

2. **Positive reinforcement**

    - **Recognizing success**: Recognize patients' progress, however modest, to boost their self-confidence.
    - **Motivation**: Maintain an encouraging attitude, even in the face of difficulties or setbacks.

- **Adapting to the environment**

Environmental adaptation is a key element in improving the quality of life, autonomy and safety of blind people. By modifying and designing living, working and public spaces, visually impaired people can navigate more easily, carry out their daily activities with confidence and participate fully in society. As a caregiver, it is essential to understand the principles and techniques of environmental adaptation to effectively support patients in this process.

Fundamentals of environmental adaptation

1. **Universal accessibility**
   Universal accessibility aims to design spaces that can be used by everyone, regardless of physical, sensory or cognitive abilities. For blind people, this means creating environments that compensate for the absence of vision through the use of other senses, notably touch, hearing and smell.

2. **Safety**
   Safety is paramount in preventing accidents and injuries. Adaptations must eliminate or minimize obstacles, potential hazards and risk situations.

3. **Autonomy**
   Adaptations must promote the patient's independence, enabling him or her to carry out daily tasks without assistance or with a minimum of help.

4. **Comfort and well-being**
   The environment must be pleasant, functional and adapted to the patient's individual preferences, thus contributing to his or her physical and mental well-being.

Home improvements

1. **Coherent spatial organization**
    - **Logical room layout**: Rooms should be arranged in such a way as to facilitate

movement. For example, the bedroom close to the bathroom.
- **Clear pathways**: Corridors and passageways must be free of obstacles such as furniture, carpets or objects on the floor.
- **Keeping things in order**: Always put things in their place so that the patient can find them easily. Avoid moving furniture without informing the patient.

2. **Tactile and visual cues**

- **Tactile markings**: Use rumble strips or textured surfaces to mark changes in level, stairs or intersections.
- **Braille or embossed labelling**: mark switches, appliances, medicine bottles or household products with tactile labels.
- **Wall guides**: Install handrails or rails to help patients move around safely.

3. **Suitable lighting**

- **For visually impaired patients**: Provide strong, uniform, glare-free lighting to improve visual perception. Use color contrasts to distinguish objects or areas.
- **Lighting control**: Install easily accessible switches, possibly with voice commands or motion detectors.

4. **Safe and functional kitchen**

- **Utensil organization**: Store kitchen utensils in an orderly fashion, using specific dividers or racks.
- **Food labelling**: Use tactile labels to identify food products, spices or condiments.

- **Adapted appliances**: Opt for appliances with tactile controls, audible signals or raised markings.
- **Safety**: Install safety devices such as gas fuses, smoke detectors and accessible fire extinguishers.

5. **Secure bathroom**

    - **Non-slip mats**: Use non-slip mats in the bath or shower, and on the floor.
    - **Grab bars**: Install grab bars near bathtubs, showers and toilets.
    - **Adapted faucets**: Choose single-lever or infrared-sensing faucets for ease of use.
    - **Tactile markers**: Mark hot/cold positions on taps with tactile symbols.

6. **Comfortable bedroom**

    - **Simple layout**: position the bed so that there's enough room to move around. Keep bedside tables within easy reach.
    - **Accessible storage**: Use easy-to-open cupboards and drawers, with organization systems for clothes.

Designing public spaces

1. **Accessible signage**

    - **Braille and raised signs**: Provide tactile information on orientation signs, room numbers or emergency indications.
    - **Audible announcements**: Install voice announcement systems in public transport, elevators or public buildings to provide information on stops, floors or directions.

2. **Safe pathways**

    - **Pedometer strips**: Use specially textured strips to guide blind people along sidewalks, station platforms or in shopping malls.
    - **Color contrasts**: For the visually impaired, use high contrasts between walls, floors and obstacles to facilitate perception.

3. **Transport accessibility**

    - **Adapted buses and trains**: Provide audible stop announcements, priority seating and access ramps.
    - **Audible pedestrian lights**: Install audible signals at crosswalks to indicate when it's safe to cross.

4. **Service accessibility**

    - **Adapted counters**: Offer counters with agents trained to help blind people, with documents available in Braille or audio format.
    - **Accessible websites**: Ensure that public service and corporate websites comply with digital accessibility standards, enabling the use of screen readers.

Using technology to adapt the environment

1. **Home automation and smart homes**

    - **Voice commands**: use voice assistants (like Amazon Alexa, Google Assistant) to control lighting, heating, appliances or security systems.
    - **Automation**: Program routines to automate certain daily tasks, such as opening shutters or turning on lights.

2. **Mobile applications and connected devices**

    - **Interior orientation applications**: Use applications that help you navigate inside buildings by providing voice instructions.
    - **Bluetooth beacons**: Install beacons that send information to the patient's smartphone to help them find their way around.

3. **Security and surveillance**

    - **Alert systems**: Install connected smoke, carbon monoxide or gas leak detectors, which emit audible signals and send notifications to the patient or family.
    - **Cameras with voice assistance**: For visually impaired patients, use cameras that describe what they see or zoom in on objects.

Involving patients in adapting their environment

1. **Individual needs assessment**

    - **Patient consultation**: Discuss with the patient to understand his or her needs, preferences and lifestyle habits.
    - **Professional assessment**: Call in occupational therapists or accessibility specialists to carry out a thorough assessment.

2. **Active participation**

    - **Choice of equipment** : Involve the patient in the choice of equipment, materials or technologies to be used.
    - **Equipment training**: Ensure that the patient is trained and comfortable with new installations or technological devices.

3. **Continuous adaptation**

   - **Regular reassessment**: Periodically review accommodations to ensure they continue to meet the patient's needs, especially if there are changes in their condition or abilities.
   - **Flexibility**: Be ready to adjust or modify layouts according to patient feedback.

The caregiver's role in adapting the environment

1. **Awareness and advice**

   - **Inform the patient and family**: Explain the importance of adapting the environment and possible solutions.
   - **Suggest practical ideas**: Suggest simple, effective layouts based on observation of the patient's needs.

2. **Working with professionals**

   - **Coordination with occupational therapists**: Work closely together to implement design recommendations.
   - **Communication with the care team**: sharing information on adaptations made and the patient's needs.

3. **Training and support**

   - **Help in using new equipment**: Accompany patients as they learn how to use installed devices.
   - **Follow-up**: Monitor the effectiveness of the facilities and report any problems or adjustments.

Raising awareness among family and community members

1. **Educating family and friends**

   - **Involvement in accommodation**: Encourage family involvement in the accommodation process to ensure consistency and ongoing support.
   - **Training**: Providing information on how to help patients while respecting their autonomy.

2. **Promoting accessibility in the community**

   - **Awareness-raising**: Participate in awareness-raising initiatives to promote the accessibility of public spaces and services.
   - **Commitment**: Encourage local institutions to adopt inclusive policies and practices.

Personal care

Personal care is a fundamental aspect of care for blind people. It encompasses all activities related to hygiene, dressing, eating and self-presentation. For blind patients, these daily tasks can present additional challenges due to vision loss. As a caregiver, your role is crucial in supporting these patients in accomplishing their personal care, promoting their autonomy, ensuring their safety and respecting their dignity.

The importance of personal care for blind people

Personal care is more than just personal hygiene; it has a significant impact on a patient's physical, emotional and social well-being. A well-groomed appearance and adequate hygiene help to boost self-esteem, prevent infections and medical complications, and facilitate social integration. For blind people, maintaining an effective personal care routine is essential to preserving their independence and quality of life.

Personal care challenges faced by blind patients

1. **Guidance and coordination**

   - **Locating objects**: Finding toiletries, clothes or accessories can be difficult without visual cues.
   - **Gesture precision**: Performing tasks requiring manual precision, such as shaving, applying make-up or trimming nails, can present risks of injury.

2. **Security**

   - **Fall hazards**: In the bathroom, slippery surfaces and obstacles can lead to falls.
   - **Appliance operation**: Handling electrical appliances or sharp objects without vision can be dangerous.

3. **Self-esteem and confidence**

   - **Dependency**: The need for assistance can affect a person's sense of autonomy and dignity.
   - **Personal image**: Uncertainty about one's appearance can lead to anxiety or reluctance to participate in social activities.

The caregiver's role in personal care

1. **Promoting autonomy**

   - **Encouraging independence**: Supporting the patient to carry out tasks he or she is capable of doing alone, by offering advice and encouragement.

- **Adapting methods**: Suggest alternative techniques to facilitate personal care, such as using adapted tools or setting up structured routines.

2. **Personalized assistance**

    - **Needs assessment**: Understanding the patient's abilities and preferences to adapt assistance appropriately.
    - **Active participation**: Involve patients in decisions concerning their care, respecting their choices and pace.

3. **Ensuring safety**

    - **Risk prevention**: Identify potential hazards and implement measures to eliminate or reduce them.
    - **Careful supervision**: Supervise patients during risky tasks, while respecting their privacy.

4. **Respect for dignity and privacy**

    - **Confidentiality**: Protecting patient privacy by providing personal care in an appropriate environment.
    - **Respectful communication**: Inform the patient at every stage, ask for his or her consent and respect his or her limits.

Techniques and approaches to support personal care

1. **Space organization**

    - **Functional layout**: Arrange toiletries and clothing in an orderly, coherent fashion to make them easy to locate.

- **Tactile cues**: Use Braille labels, different textures or distinctive shapes to identify objects.

2. **Training in adapted techniques**

    - **Self-care methods**: Teach the patient safe techniques for performing tasks such as shaving, brushing teeth or applying care products.
    - **Use of technical aids**: Present tools designed to facilitate personal care, such as electric razors with protection, ergonomic nail clippers or measuring devices for liquid products.

3. **Effective communication**

    - **Clear instructions**: Provide detailed, step-by-step explanations for complex tasks.
    - **Positive feedback**: Valorize the patient's efforts and successes to boost confidence.

4. **Emotional support**

    - **Empathetic listening**: Being attentive to the patient's concerns, particularly regarding his or her appearance or difficulties.
    - **Encouraging expression**: Invite patients to share their feelings and needs, creating a climate of trust.

Assistance with specific activities

1. **Personal hygiene**

    - **Bath and shower**: Install grab bars, non-slip mats and shower seats to ensure safety. Offer pump soap dispensers for ease of use.

- **Intimate grooming**: Respect the patient's privacy, offering help only if necessary and providing verbal guidance.

2. **Dental care**

    - **Brushing teeth**: Suggest the use of electric toothbrushes with audible timers. Explain the quadrant brushing technique for complete coverage.
    - **Product identification**: Use tactile labels to distinguish toothpaste from other products.

3. **Hair care**

    - **Shampoo**: Offer pump bottles for easy dosing. Guide patients through application and rinsing.
    - **Hair styling**: Provide ergonomic combs or brushes. If patients wish to style their own hair, explain simple techniques.

4. **Clothing**

    - **Clothing organization**: Classify garments by type and color, using markers such as different-shaped pins.
    - **Choosing outfits**: Help patients coordinate their clothes by describing colors and patterns. Encourage self-expression.

5. **Nail care**

    - **Safety**: If the patient is not comfortable cutting his or her own nails, offer to do so or call in a professional.
    - **Adapted techniques**: Teaching safe nail filing methods.

6. **Shaving and make-up**

    - **Shaving**: Recommend electric razors with protective heads to avoid cuts.
    - **Make-up**: For patients wishing to wear make-up, suggest products that are easy to apply, such as lipstick pencils or eye shadow sticks.

Promoting autonomy in personal care

1. **Establishing routines**

    - **Regular schedules**: Help the patient establish a schedule for personal care, which facilitates memorization and predictability.
    - **Lists and audio guides**: Provide recordings or tactile lists of the steps to follow for certain tasks.

2. **Skills development**

    - **Practical workshops**: Organize learning sessions to perfect personal care techniques.
    - **Encouraging self-evaluation**: Invite patients to evaluate their work, for example by checking the result with their hands.

3. **Use of assistive technologies**

    - **Mobile applications**: Present applications that offer voice instructions or reminders for personal care.
    - **Connected devices**: Use talking mirrors or scales with voice synthesis.

Ensuring safety during personal care

1. **Accident prevention**

    - **Safe equipment**: Regularly check the condition of electrical appliances and replace any that are faulty.
    - **Adequate lighting**: For visually impaired patients, ensure sufficient glare-free lighting.

2. **Discreet surveillance**

    - **Attentive presence**: Being available to intervene when needed, while allowing the patient to act autonomously.
    - **Alarms and detectors**: Install devices that alert you in the event of a fall or problem, without being intrusive.

Respect for dignity and privacy

1. **Consent**

    - **Prior request**: Always ask permission before helping the patient with personal tasks.
    - **Right of refusal**: Respect the patient's choice to carry out certain tasks alone or with another person.

2. **Privacy**

    - **Discretion**: Do not divulge information concerning the patient's personal care to unauthorized third parties.
    - **Suitable environment**: Carry out care in a private area, out of sight and out of mind.

Collaboration with the interdisciplinary team

1. **Care coordination**

   - **Communication with professionals**: Working with nurses, occupational therapists and other team members to ensure coherent care.
   - **Information sharing**: Report any difficulties encountered by the patient or progress made.

2. **Continuing education**

   - **Skills updating**: Participate in training courses to learn new techniques or innovative approaches to personal care.
   - **Sharing best practice**: Discuss effective strategies for supporting patients with colleagues.

Involving family and friends

1. **Awareness**

   - **Information**: Explain to family and friends the importance of personal care for the patient's well-being.
   - **Practical advice**: Provide recommendations on how to help patients at home, while respecting their autonomy.

2. **Emotional support**

   - **Encouragement**: Encourage the family to value the patient's efforts and support him in his initiatives.
   - **Dealing with frustration**: Help loved ones understand the challenges facing the patient and adopt an empathetic attitude.

Medication management

Medication management is a crucial aspect of care for blind people. It is particularly important because of the risks associated with improper administration, such as overdosing, drug interactions or missing essential doses. For blind patients, the challenges of independent medication management are amplified by the absence of visual cues. As a caregiver, your role is fundamental in supporting these patients in organizing, understanding and safely administering their treatments, while promoting their autonomy and respecting their dignity.

The importance of safe medication management

Effective medication management ensures that the patient receives the right medication, at the right dose, at the right time and in the right way. For blind people, medication errors can have serious consequences for their health. In addition, inadequate management can lead to a loss of self-confidence, increased dependence on caregivers and a deterioration in quality of life.

Specific challenges faced by blind patients

1. **Drug identification**
    - **Packaging similarity**: Many medicines have similar packaging, making it difficult to distinguish them by sight.
    - **Lack of tactile labels**: Essential information, such as the name of the drug, dosage or expiration date, is usually printed in small type, inaccessible to blind people.
    - **Similar shapes and textures**: tablets, capsules or liquids can be difficult to distinguish by touch.

2. **Organization and storage**

    ○ **Dose confusion**: Without a proper organizational system, it's easy to mix up medications or take the wrong dose.
    ○ **Managing schedules**: remembering the precise times to take each medication without a visual cue can be complex.

3. **Reading instructions**

    ○ **Limited access to user manuals**: User manuals are rarely available in Braille or audio format.
    ○ **Understanding treatment changes**: Changes prescribed by the doctor may not be communicated in an accessible way.

The caregiver's role in medication management

1. **Ensuring safety**

    ○ **Medication verification**: Confirm that the patient is taking the right medication, at the right dose, at the right time.
    ○ **Error prevention**: Implement systems to avoid mix-ups, such as the use of adapted pillboxes.

2. **Promoting autonomy**

    ○ **Patient education**: Teaching people how to manage their medication independently.
    ○ **Use of assistive technologies**: Introduce devices or applications that facilitate medication management.

3. **Effective communication**
    - **Clear explanations**: Provide understandable information on drugs, their effects and administration instructions.
    - **Active listening**: Encourage patients to express any concerns or questions they may have about their treatment.

4. **Coordination with the medical team**
    - **Transmission of information**: Communicate with nurses, pharmacists and physicians to ensure that the patient receives appropriate care.
    - **Updating treatments**: Find out about prescription changes and explain them to the patient.

Techniques and strategies to support medication management

1. **Drug organization**
    - **Suitable pillboxes**: Use weekly or daily pillboxes with separate compartments for each time of day. Some models have tactile markings or raised color codes.
    - **Labeling in Braille or large print**: Mark medication boxes with tactile labels indicating the name of the drug and dosage.
    - **Tactile coding systems**: Use rubber bands, embossed shapes or stickers with different textures to differentiate medicines.

2. **Use of assistive technologies**
    - **Mobile applications**: Offer applications that remind you when to take your medication,

provide voice-activated drug information, or allow you to scan barcodes for audio descriptions.
- **Talking devices**: Use electronic pillboxes with audible alarms or devices that announce the name of the medication and the dose.
- **Barcode readers**: Devices that read out information from drug labels.

3. **Patient education**

    - **Explanation of treatments**: Provide detailed information on each drug, its usefulness, possible side effects and precautions to be taken.
    - **Training in management techniques**: Teaching how to organize medications, use assistive devices and recognize different medications by touch or smell if possible.

4. **Securing the environment**

    - **Dedicated space**: Create a specific, easily accessible and coherently organized area for storing medications.
    - **Disposal of expired medications**: Help patients identify and dispose of expired medications to avoid mix-ups.

Ensuring safety and compliance

1. **Error prevention**

    - **Double-checking**: Encourage patients to double-check each medication before taking it, using labeling systems or talking devices.

- **Discreet monitoring**: If necessary, supervise the taking of medication, while respecting the patient's autonomy.

2. **Renewal management**

    - **Anticipation**: Help patients monitor remaining quantities and plan refills in good time.
    - **Coordination with the pharmacy**: Facilitate communication with the pharmacist for orders, deliveries or packaging adaptations.

3. **Monitoring side effects**

    - **Careful observation**: watch for signs of adverse reactions or allergic reactions.
    - **Communication with physician**: Report any abnormalities or concerns regarding treatment.

Encouraging patient autonomy

1. **Building trust**

    - **Positive reinforcement**: Praise the patient's self-management of medication, boosting their confidence in their abilities.
    - **Progressive management**: Start with simple tasks and gradually increase the patient's responsibility for managing his or her medication.

2. **Adapting to individual preferences**

    - **Personalizing methods**: Adapting strategies to the patient's habits, cognitive abilities and preferences.
    - **Flexibility**: Be ready to modify approaches if certain methods are not suitable for the patient.

Involving family and friends

1. **Collaborative support**
   - **Informing family members**: Explain to family members the medication management systems in place.
   - **Active participation**: Encourage family and friends to support the patient, while respecting his or her autonomy.

2. **Caregiver training**
   - **Assistance techniques**: Train family carers in the methods used to provide consistent assistance.
   - **Risk awareness**: Inform about the importance of medication safety and the potential consequences of errors.

Collaboration with healthcare professionals

1. **Pharmacists**
   - **Suitable packaging**: Ask your pharmacist to supply medicines in easy-to-handle packaging, with labels in Braille or large print if possible.
   - **Clear information**: Ensure that the patient receives understandable explanations about new medications or changes in treatment.

2. **Nurses and doctors**
   - **Care planning**: Participate in team meetings to coordinate care and share relevant information.
   - **Therapeutic education**: Working together to provide patients with comprehensive education on their disease and treatment.

Ethical and deontological compliance

1. **Privacy**

    - **Data protection**: Ensuring that patient medical information is kept securely and shared only with the professionals concerned.

2. **Informed consent**

    - **Transparent information**: Providing patients with all the information they need to make informed decisions about their health and treatment.
    - **Respect for decisions**: Honor the patient's choices, even if they differ from recommendations, while ensuring that he or she understands the implications.

Continuing training for nurses' aides

1. **Updating knowledge**

    - **New technologies**: Keep abreast of innovations in assistive devices for medication management.
    - **Regulations**: Know the laws and guidelines concerning the handling of medicines.

2. **Skills development**

    - **Workshops and training**: Participate in training programs to improve skills in medication management and patient education.
    - **Sharing experiences**: Exchange with other professionals to learn best practices and solutions to common challenges.

Chapter 5

Psychological and social support

Recognizing the signs of emotional distress

Emotional distress is a natural reaction to difficult, stressful or traumatic situations. For people who are blind, the daily challenges of vision loss can accentuate this type of distress. As a caregiver, it is essential to know how to identify the signs of emotional distress in order to provide appropriate support, prevent psychological complications and promote the patient's overall well-being.

Understanding emotional distress in blind people

Blindness can have a profound impact on a person's life, affecting not only their ability to interact with the physical world, but also their emotional and psychological state. Feelings of loss, frustration, isolation or fear are common and can, if left unaddressed, lead to more serious disorders such as depression or anxiety.

Blind people can experience :

- **A sense of loss**: vision loss is often associated with bereavement, with feelings similar to those experienced when losing a loved one.
- **Daily frustrations**: Difficulties in accomplishing previously simple tasks can lead to anger and frustration.
- **Social isolation**: Blindness can limit social interaction, leading to feelings of loneliness.
- **Fear of the future**: Uncertainty about one's ability to live independently or carry out personal projects can generate anxiety.

Signs and symptoms of emotional distress

It's important to recognize that emotional distress can manifest itself in different, often subtle, ways. Here are the main signs to watch out for:

1. **Sudden or persistent mood swings**

    - **Sadness or depression**: The patient may appear downcast, cry frequently or express feelings of despair.
    - **Irritability or anger**: Excessive reactions to minor situations, impatience or unusual outbursts of anger.
    - **Anxiety**: Excessive worry, nervousness, fear for no apparent reason.

2. **Social withdrawal**

    - **Isolation**: The patient avoids interaction with others, refuses visits or social activities.
    - **Loss of interest**: Decreased involvement in activities previously enjoyed.

3. **Changes in sleep and appetite patterns**

    - **Insomnia or hypersomnia**: difficulty falling asleep, frequent awakenings, excessive sleep.
    - **Fluctuating appetite**: Loss or gain of appetite, which can lead to weight fluctuations.

4. **Reduced energy and motivation**

    - **Constant fatigue**: Feeling tired despite rest.
    - **Difficulty concentrating**: Memory problems, difficulty making decisions.

5. **Verbal expressions of distress**

    ○ **Negative self-talk**: the patient devalues himself, expresses feelings of worthlessness or guilt.
    ○ **Suicidal ideation**: references to death, desire to stop living, concrete plans to harm oneself.

6. **Unusual behavior**

    ○ **Psychomotor agitation**: Nervous movements, inability to stay put.
    ○ **Slowness** : Slowness of movement or speech.

7. **Physical signs**

    ○ **Headaches, pain**: No apparent medical cause.
    ○ **Digestive problems**: nausea, stress-related intestinal disorders.

Factors contributing to emotional distress

Several factors can exacerbate emotional distress in blind people:

- **Recency of vision loss**: Recent blindness is often more difficult to accept.
- **Lack of social support**: Lack of family or friends can increase feelings of isolation.
- **Financial difficulties**: Economic constraints can add stress.
- **Medical co-morbidities**: The presence of other health problems can complicate the situation.

The caregiver's role in identifying emotional distress

As a caregiver, you're often on the front line of observing changes in the patient. Your role includes:

1. **Careful observation**
    - **Watch for signs**: Be alert to changes in behavior, mood or physical health.
    - **Record variations**: Keep a log of observations to detect trends or patterns.

2. **Open communication**
    - **Active listening**: Take the time to listen to the patient without judgment, showing empathy.
    - **Open-ended questions**: Encourage patients to express their feelings by asking questions such as "How are you feeling today?".

3. **Creating a safe environment**
    - **Mutual trust**: Establish a relationship based on respect and confidentiality.
    - **Assurance of support**: Reassuring the patient that he or she is not alone and that help is available.

4. **Appropriate response**
    - **Validating feelings**: Recognize the patient's emotions as legitimate.
    - **Avoid minimization**: Don't say things like "It's nothing" or "Everything will be fine" without taking concrete action.

5. **Coordination with healthcare professionals**
    - **Reporting**: Inform nurses, doctors or psychologists of worrying signs.
    - **Follow-up**: Collaborate to implement appropriate interventions.

Possible interventions to help the patient

1. **Emotional support**
   - **Presence**: Being there for the patient, even in silence.
   - **Soothing activities**: Offer relaxing activities such as listening to music, reading aloud or relaxation exercises.

2. **Encouraging self-expression**
   - **Support groups**: Refer patients to discussion groups or associations.
   - **Therapy**: Suggest a consultation with a psychologist or psychiatrist.

3. **Promoting autonomy**
   - **Skills development**: Helping patients acquire new skills to boost their confidence.
   - **Realistic goals**: Set achievable goals with the patient to give them a sense of accomplishment.

4. **Family involvement**
   - **Communication with loved ones**: With the patient's consent, involve the family in providing emotional support.
   - **Education**: Inform loved ones about emotional distress and how they can help.

Preventing emotional distress

- **Preventive education**: Inform patients about possible emotional reactions to vision loss.
- **Social activities**: Encourage participation in community activities to avoid isolation.

- **Self-care**: Promote healthy lifestyle habits, such as a balanced diet, appropriate physical activity and adequate sleep.
- **Stress management**: Teaching relaxation or meditation techniques.

When to seek professional help

If you observe signs of severe or persistent emotional distress, it's crucial to seek the intervention of mental health professionals. The following situations require immediate attention:

- **Suicidal ideation or self-destructive behavior**
- **Rapid deterioration in emotional state**
- **Inability to perform daily activities**
- **Hallucinations or delusions**

Psychological support techniques

Psychological support for blind people is an essential dimension of comprehensive care. Blindness, whether congenital or acquired, can present significant emotional and psychological challenges. As a caregiver, it is essential to master the techniques of psychological support to help patients adapt and improve their quality of life. This support is based on an empathetic approach, adapted communication and the use of specific therapeutic strategies to help patients overcome the emotional obstacles associated with their condition.

Understanding the psychological impact of blindness

Vision loss can lead to a multitude of emotional reactions, including :

- **Shock and denial**: Especially in cases of acquired blindness, patients may find it hard to accept the reality of their situation.
- **Anger and frustration**: Functional limitations can provoke anger towards oneself or others.
- **Sadness and depression**: A sense of loss can lead to depression, with symptoms such as hopelessness or loss of interest in activities.
- **Anxiety**: Fear of the future, the unknown or new situations can generate anxiety.
- **Social isolation**: difficulty participating in social activities can reinforce feelings of loneliness.

Recognizing these reactions is the first step in providing appropriate psychological support.

Fundamental principles of psychological support

1. **Establishing a relationship of trust**
   Trust is the cornerstone of all psychological support. To build it :
   - **Constant presence**: Be available and show commitment to the patient's well-being.
   - **Respect and non-judgment**: Welcome the patient's feelings and thoughts without criticism.
   - **Confidentiality**: Assuring patients that shared information remains confidential.

2. **Active and empathetic listening**
   - **Total attention**: Concentrate fully on the patient during exchanges.
   - **Reformulation**: Repeating in your own words what the patient has said, to show your understanding.
   - **Emotional validation**: Acknowledging the patient's feelings as legitimate.

3. **Adapted communication**

    - **Clarity and simplicity**: Use accessible language, avoid medical jargon.
    - **Open-ended questions**: Encourage patients to express themselves more fully by asking non-directive questions.
    - **Patience**: Give patients time to formulate their thoughts without rushing them.

4. **Promoting autonomy**

    - **Encourage participation**: Involve patients in decisions concerning their care.
    - **Positive reinforcement**: Emphasize progress and efforts made.
    - **Skills development**: Helping patients acquire new skills to boost their self-confidence.

Specific psychological support techniques

1. **Person-centred approach**
Inspired by Carl Rogers, this approach focuses on :

    - **Deep empathy**: Connecting with the patient's experiences.
    - **Congruence**: Being authentic in interactions.
    - **The unconditional positive gaze**: Accepting the patient unconditionally.

2. **Cognitive behavioral therapy (CBT)**
Although the caregiver is not a psychotherapist, he or she can use certain principles of CBT to help the patient :

    - **Identify negative thoughts**: Recognize thought patterns that generate stress or anxiety.

- **Restructuring beliefs**: Encouraging a more realistic, positive outlook.
- **Develop coping strategies**: Teach stress management techniques such as deep breathing and muscle relaxation.

3. **Stress management techniques**

    - **Relaxation**: offer guided relaxation exercises to reduce tension.
    - **Mindfulness**: Encourage the patient to focus on the present moment, accepting sensations and emotions without judgment.
    - **Adapted physical activity**: Promote activities such as walking or yoga, which can improve mood and reduce anxiety.

4. **Peer support**

    - **Support groups**: Refer patients to groups where they can share their experiences with other blind people.
    - **Mentoring**: Facilitating contact with individuals who have overcome similar challenges.

5. **Art therapy and creative expression**

    - **Music, writing, sculpture**: Encourage forms of expression that enable patients to communicate their emotions non-verbally.
    - **Creative workshops**: Organize or suggest activities that stimulate creativity and promote well-being.

Support in coming to terms with blindness

Helping patients accept their condition is a delicate process that requires :

- **Time and patience**: Understand that acceptance is a step that can take time.
- **Ongoing support**: Being present during difficult times, offering an attentive ear.
- **Information**: Provide resources on blindness, assistive technologies, rights and opportunities.
- **Emphasizing abilities**: Focusing on the patient's skills and talents rather than their limitations.

Dealing with difficult emotions

1. **Anger and frustration**

    - **Constructive channeling**: Encourage the expression of anger through healthy means, such as exercise or discussion.
    - **Relaxation techniques**: Teach patients to recognize signs of tension and use methods to calm themselves.

2. **Sadness and depression**

    - **Recognizing the signs**: Be alert to the symptoms of depression, such as despair or loss of interest.
    - **Encouraging activity**: Motivating the patient to take part in pleasant or stimulating activities.
    - **Referral to professionals**: If necessary, refer the patient to a psychologist or psychiatrist.

3. **Anxiety and fear**

    - **Gradual exposure**: Help the patient to gradually confront anxiety-provoking situations.
    - **Relaxation training**: Teaching techniques to reduce the physical symptoms of anxiety.

- **Planning**: Help patients prepare for stressful situations by developing strategies in advance.

Strengthening social support

- **Family and friends**: Encourage patients to maintain and strengthen their ties with loved ones.
- **Community involvement**: Encourage people to join clubs, associations or social activities.
- **Communication**: Helping patients express their needs and feelings to those around them.

Self-care and empowerment

- **Health education**: Informing patients about the importance of taking care of their physical and mental health.
- **Goal setting**: Work with the patient to set realistic, achievable goals.
- **Autonomy**: Encourage the use of assistive technologies and techniques that promote independence.

Collaboration with mental health professionals

- **Care coordination**: working as a team with psychologists, psychiatrists and social workers.
- **Continuity of support** : Regular, consistent follow-up.
- **Information sharing**: Communicate relevant observations while respecting confidentiality.

Continuing training for nurses' aides

- **Skills development**: Participate in training courses on psychological support techniques.
- **Supervision**: Benefit from the guidance of experienced professionals to improve your practice.
- **Self-reflection**: Regularly evaluate your approach and look for ways to improve it.

Promoting social integration

The social integration of blind people is a major challenge that goes beyond the medical framework to touch on human, cultural and societal dimensions. It aims to enable individuals affected by blindness to participate fully in community life, enjoying the same rights, opportunities and responsibilities as other citizens. As a caregiver, your role is essential in fostering this integration, by supporting the patient not only physically and psychologically, but also by helping him or her to overcome the social and environmental barriers that can hinder active participation in society.

Understanding the challenges of social integration

Blind people can face various obstacles that limit their social participation:

- **Prejudice and stereotypes**: Preconceived ideas about blindness can lead to paternalistic attitudes, discrimination or exclusion.
- **Limited accessibility**: The inaccessibility of public places, transport, information and technology can restrict autonomy and mobility.
- **Social isolation**: Difficulty establishing and maintaining social relationships can lead to feelings of loneliness and isolation.
- **Barriers to employment and education**: Barriers in the world of work and education can limit opportunities for personal and professional development.

The role of the caregiver in promoting social integration

As a caregiver, you can positively influence a patient's social integration by taking a proactive, holistic approach:

1. **Promoting autonomy and self-confidence**

    - **Skills development**: Helping patients acquire the skills they need to manage their daily lives, using assistive technologies, mobility techniques and adapted communication methods.
    - **Positive reinforcement**: Encourage patients by recognizing their successes, thus boosting their self-esteem and motivation to become socially involved.
    - **Support for decision-making**: Involve patients in decisions that concern them, respecting their choices and promoting their autonomy.

2. **Facilitating access to resources and opportunities**

    - **Rights information**: Informing patients of their rights in terms of accessibility, education, employment and civic participation.
    - **Referral to appropriate services**: Connect the patient with available associations, training centers, employment services and support programs.
    - **Administrative support**: Helping patients with administrative procedures to access social benefits, financial aid and support services.

3. **Raising awareness in the community**

    - **Loved ones' education**: Inform family and friends about blindness, the patient's abilities and how to support them appropriately.
    - **Promoting inclusive attitudes**: Encourage those around you to adopt respectful behaviors, avoid stereotypes and encourage the patient's active participation.
    - **Participation in awareness-raising activities**: Involve the patient in activities aimed at

informing the public about blindness and promoting inclusion.

4. **Facilitating social participation**

    - **Encourage social activities**: Motivate patients to take part in clubs, associations, cultural or sporting events adapted to their interests.
    - **Leisure support**: Help patients discover and engage in recreational activities that promote social interaction, such as music, theater, sports or volunteer work.
    - **Personalized support**: If necessary, accompany patients when they first participate, to provide support and reassurance.

5. **Promoting universal accessibility**

    - **Environmental planning**: Working with institutions to improve the accessibility of public spaces, transport and services.
    - **Use of technology**: Encourage the adoption of accessible technologies that facilitate communication, information and social participation.
    - **Advocacy for inclusion**: Support initiatives aimed at strengthening public policies in favor of accessibility and inclusion for people with disabilities.

Strategies for overcoming barriers to social integration

1. **Fighting prejudice**

    - **Education and awareness**: Organize or participate in workshops, conferences or

awareness campaigns to deconstruct stereotypes associated with blindness.
- **Highlighting success stories**: Share stories of blind people who have succeeded in various fields, to inspire the patient and change social perceptions.

2. **Strengthening social skills**
   - **Developing communication skills**: Helping patients improve their verbal communication, emotional expression and active listening skills.
   - **Managing social interactions**: Teach strategies for approaching new people, participating in conversations and handling awkward social situations.

3. **Psychological support**
   - **Therapeutic support**: If the patient is experiencing social anxiety, depression or other emotional difficulties, refer them to mental health professionals.
   - **Peer support groups**: Encourage participation in groups where patients can share their experiences and receive support from people in similar situations.

4. **Facilitating access to education and employment**
   - **Career guidance**: Help patients identify their interests and skills, and explore training and career options.
   - **Job search assistance**: Helping patients to write CVs, prepare for interviews and find professional opportunities.
   - **Adapting work environments**: Working with employers to provide reasonable

accommodations that enable the patient to work effectively.

Working with key players

1. **Specialized associations and organizations**

   - **Networking**: Put the patient in touch with blind people's associations that offer resources, activities and support.
   - **Community involvement**: Encourage patient involvement in community initiatives, thereby strengthening their sense of belonging.

2. **Educational institutions**

   - **Adaptation of educational materials**: Work with schools or training centers to ensure that educational materials are accessible.
   - **Academic support**: Facilitate access to tutors, teaching aids or assistive technologies to support academic success.

3. **Employers and the workplace**

   - **Raising awareness among employers**: Promoting the advantages of hiring blind people and informing them about possible accommodations.
   - **Professional mentoring**: Encourage mentoring programs where the patient can be guided by experienced professionals.

Importance of empowerment

Empowerment is a process by which patients acquire the confidence, skills and means to control their lives and exercise their rights. By promoting empowerment, you help patients to become active players in their own social integration:

- **Building resilience**: Encouraging patients to overcome obstacles and persevere in the face of challenges.
- **Awareness of rights**: Inform patients of their legal rights and how to assert them.
- **Encouraging self-advocacy**: Supporting patients' ability to express their needs, make decisions and actively participate in processes that affect them.

Promoting an inclusive society

Beyond individual support, it is important to contribute to building a society that values diversity and inclusion:

- **Advocacy for equality**: Support legislative and policy initiatives aimed at eliminating discrimination and promoting equal opportunities.
- **Public education**: Participate in educational programs that raise public awareness of the issues surrounding the inclusion of blind people.
- **Cross-sector collaboration**: Working with governments, non-governmental organizations, businesses and communities to create accessible and welcoming environments for all.

Chapter 6

Rehabilitation and re-education

Vision rehabilitation programs

Vision rehabilitation is an essential process designed to help people with visual impairment maximize the use of their residual vision, develop compensatory skills and improve their quality of life. For blind or visually impaired patients, these programs offer tools and strategies to overcome daily challenges, promote independence and facilitate social integration. As a caregiver, it is important to understand the role and benefits of vision rehabilitation programs in order to effectively support patients on this journey.

Understanding vision rehabilitation

Vision rehabilitation is aimed at people with significantly impaired vision, whether complete blindness or partial visual impairment. The causes can be varied: eye diseases (such as age-related macular degeneration, glaucoma, diabetic retinopathy), trauma or congenital conditions. The main aim of vision rehabilitation is to help patients make the most of their remaining visual capacities, and develop strategies to compensate for their limitations.

The objectives of vision rehabilitation programs

1. **Improve visual efficiency**: optimize the use of residual vision through specific exercises and techniques.

2. **Develop compensatory skills**: Learn to use other senses, such as touch and hearing, to supplement vision.

3. **Facilitate autonomy**: Acquire the skills to carry out activities of daily living independently.

4. **Support psychological adaptation**: Help patients accept their condition, manage associated emotions and maintain a positive attitude.

5. **Promoting social and professional integration**: Preparing patients to take an active part in social life and, if possible, to resume or maintain a professional activity.

Professionals involved in vision rehabilitation

Vision rehabilitation is an interdisciplinary process involving several healthcare professionals:

- **Ophthalmologists**: They diagnose visual disorders, assess residual vision and refer patients to the appropriate rehabilitation services.

- **Orthoptists**: Specialized in visual rehabilitation, they set up exercise programs to improve visual abilities.

- **Occupational therapists**: They help patients adapt their environment and develop strategies for carrying out daily activities.

- **Locomotion instructors**: They teach safe movement techniques, including the use of the white cane and orientation in different environments.

- **Psychologists**: They help patients adapt emotionally to vision loss.

- **Vision aid technicians**: They advise on optical and technological devices that can improve vision or compensate for its loss.

Techniques and methods used

1. **Visual stimulation exercises**
   Orthoptists offer exercises to improve fixation, eye tracking, hand-eye coordination and visual perception.

These exercises are adapted to the patient's abilities and may include:

- **Light stimulation**: using light sources to stimulate the retina.
- **Visual games**: Fun activities to work on shape, color and contrast discrimination.

2. **Use of optical aids**

    - **Magnifiers and telescopic systems**: to enlarge images and make it easier to read or observe distant objects.
    - **Specific filters and glasses**: to improve contrast and reduce glare.

3. **Assistive technologies**

    - **Screen magnification software**: To make computers easier to use.
    - Text-to-speech: Read text aloud.
    - **Adapted mobile applications**: For navigation, text and object recognition.

4. **Braille learning**
For patients with severe vision loss, learning Braille enables them to read and write, thus promoting access to education and information.

5. **Orientation and mobility techniques**

    - **Using the white cane**: Learn to detect obstacles and move around safely.

- **Spatial orientation**: Develop auditory, tactile and olfactory cues for navigating the environment.

6. **Adapting to the environment**

    - **Home layout**: logical organization of spaces, installation of tactile markers, improved lighting for the visually impaired.
    - **Accessible signage**: Use of Braille or raised markings in public places.

7. **Sensory substitution techniques**

    - **Tactile and auditory education**: Developing sensitivity in other senses to compensate for vision loss.
    - **Substitution devices**: For example, devices that convert images into sound.

The role of the caregiver in vision rehabilitation programs

1. **Support in setting up exercises**

    - **Coaching**: Help the patient carry out the exercises prescribed by the orthoptist, ensuring that they are carried out correctly and regularly.
    - **Motivation**: Encourage patients, reward their progress and maintain their commitment to the program.

2. **Assistance in using technical aids**

    - **Hands-on training**: Explain how the devices work, help set them up and maintain them.

- **Integration into daily life**: Encourage the use of aids in everyday activities to reinforce independence.

3. **Adapting to the environment**

    - **Concrete improvements**: Participate in the organization of the patient's living space according to the recommendations of occupational therapists.
    - **Safety**: Identify and eliminate obstacles or potential hazards.

4. **Psychological support**

    - **Active listening**: listening to the patient's concerns, offering an empathetic ear.
    - **Encouragement**: Help patients overcome frustrations, boost their confidence in their abilities.

5. **Coordination with interdisciplinary team**

    - **Effective communication**: Pass on relevant observations to other professionals involved.
    - **Participation in follow-up meetings**: Help evaluate progress and adjust the program.

Benefits for patients

1. **Improved visual function**

    - **Optimization of residual vision**: improved visual acuity, enhanced contrast and color perception.

- **Reduced visual fatigue**: Thanks to adapted techniques, patients can perform visual tasks for longer, with less effort.

2. **Increased autonomy**

    - **Independence in daily activities**: reading, writing, cooking, managing medication, getting around.
    - **Social participation**: Involvement in community, cultural or professional activities.

3. **Improved quality of life**

    - **Emotional well-being**: Reduced anxiety and depression, increased self-esteem.
    - **Personal satisfaction**: A sense of accomplishment and control over one's life.

The limits and challenges of vision rehabilitation programs

- **Patient motivation**: The success of the program depends on the patient's commitment. Psychological obstacles may hinder participation.
- **Variability of results**: Progress may be slow or limited, depending on the nature and severity of the visual impairment.
- **Accessibility of resources**: Rehabilitation services may be limited depending on the region, and some devices may be expensive.

- **Individual adaptation**: Every patient is unique. Programs must be personalized, which requires in-depth assessment and regular follow-up.

Learning Braille and other communication systems

Access to communication is a fundamental right that promotes individual autonomy, education, social integration and well-being. For blind people, Braille and other adapted communication systems play an essential role in achieving these goals. Learning Braille not only enables people to read and write, but also to develop independence in information management, education and working life. As a caregiver, it is crucial to understand the importance of these systems, to support the patient in learning them, and to encourage their use on a daily basis.

The importance of Braille in the lives of blind people

Braille is a tactile writing system invented by Louis Braille in the XIXe century. It is based on combinations of six raised dots that represent letters, numbers, punctuation and even mathematical and musical symbols. Braille is much more than a simple means of reading; it is a tool for emancipation that opens the doors to education, culture and information.

1. **Access to education and culture**
   Learning Braille enables blind people to read books, newspapers, musical scores and educational documents. This encourages independent learning, the pursuit of higher education and access to a wide range of knowledge.

2. **Developing independence**
   The ability to read and write in Braille reinforces independence in managing everyday tasks, such as taking notes, managing appointments or reading Braille labels on products.

3. **Professional integration**
   Mastering Braille can be an asset in the world of work, particularly in fields requiring precise management of written information. It can open up professional opportunities and facilitate access to qualified positions.

4. **Personal communication**
   Braille enables you to exchange written messages with other blind people, keep a diary or correspond with friends and family.

Braille learning process

Learning Braille is a process that takes time, patience and regular practice. It can be undertaken at any age, whether blindness is congenital or acquired.

1. **Initial assessment**
   Before starting, an assessment of the patient's needs and abilities is carried out by specialized professionals, such as Braille teachers or visual impairment rehabilitators. This assessment takes into account :
   - **Tactile sensitivity**: to check the ability to distinguish points in relief.
   - **Motivation and personal goals**: Understanding patient expectations.
   - **Cognitive skills**: Ensuring that the patient can assimilate the necessary concepts.

2. **Teaching methods**
Braille instruction is tailored to the patient's individual needs and may include :

- **Integral Braille**: Learn the 64 possible combinations of the six dots representing each letter and symbol.
- **Abbreviated braille**: Use of contractions and abbreviations to speed up reading and writing, often taught after full braille has been mastered.

3. Teaching methods include:

- **Tactile exercises**: Develop finger sensitivity and point recognition.
- **Reading practice**: Start with simple words, then move on to more complex sentences and texts.
- **Braille writing**: using the tablet and punch, then the Perkins machine or electronic devices.

4. **Teaching aids**
Several tools are used to facilitate learning:

- **Tablets and punches**: For Braille handwriting.
- **Braille typewriters**: Like the Perkins machine, which facilitates rapid writing.
- **Educational tactile media**: Raised letters, educational games, tactile cards.
- **Software and applications** : Interactive programs for learning Braille on computer or tablet.

5. **Professional supervision**
Apprenticeships are generally supervised by :

- **Specialized teachers**: trained to teach Braille to children and adults.

- **Rehabilitation centers**: offering comprehensive programs including Braille and other skills.
- **Associations and organizations**: offering courses, resources and support.

Other suitable communication systems

In addition to Braille, there are other systems and technologies that facilitate communication and access to information for blind people.

1. **Voice assistance technologies**
   - **Screen readers**: Software that converts on-screen text into text-to-speech, for use on computers and smartphones.
   - **Voice assistants**: devices like Siri, Alexa or Google Assistant, which respond to voice commands to perform various tasks.
   - **Mobile applications**: Many applications are designed to help recognize objects, text or colors using the smartphone's camera.

2. **Electronic Braille displays**
   These devices, also known as Braille displays, connect to a computer or smartphone and translate the displayed text into Braille in real time. They enable more discreet interaction and can be essential for tasks requiring silent or accurate reading.

3. **Alternative tactile scoring systems**
   - **Moon**: A simplified tactile system using shapes that are easier to distinguish than Braille, sometimes used for people with tactile discrimination difficulties.

- **Tactile code systems**: Use customized symbols or codes to mark objects, documents or locations.

4. **Haptic communication**

    - **Haptic techniques**: Using touch to transmit information, such as vibratory signals or tactile movements on the skin.
    - **Haptic devices**: Technologies that provide tactile feedback, such as vibrating watches for notifications or tactile navigation devices.

5. **Tactile sign language**
For deaf-blind people, sign language can be adapted in tactile mode, where the signs are made in the receiver's hand.

The caregiver's role in learning and using communication systems

1. **Emotional and motivational support**

    - **Encouraging the patient**: Provide constant support to maintain motivation, especially in the face of initial difficulties.
    - **Valuing progress**: Recognize and celebrate every step forward, no matter how small, to boost self-confidence.

2. **Practical assistance**

    - **Help with organization**: facilitate access to classes, manage schedules, liaise with teachers.
    - **Exercise participation**: If appropriate, practice with the patient to reinforce learning.

- **Adapting the environment**: Install the necessary equipment, organize the space to facilitate practice.

3. **Coordination with professionals**

    - **Regular communication**: Exchange with teachers and specialists to monitor progress and adapt support.
    - **Participation in meetings**: Attend team meetings to contribute to personalized action plans.

4. **Promoting autonomy**

    - **Encouraging independence**: Encouraging the patient to use communication systems in daily activities.
    - **Facilitate access to resources**: provide information on Braille libraries, audio books and accessible websites.

5. **Raising awareness**

    - **Inform family and friends**: Explain the importance of Braille and other systems to encourage their support.
    - **Encourage patience and understanding**: Help those around you to understand the patient's challenges and efforts.

Braille learning challenges and solutions

1. **Sensory challenges**

    - **Reduced tactile sensitivity**: In some people, finger sensitivity may be insufficient, making it difficult to discriminate points.

- **Solution**: Specific exercises to improve sensitivity, or the use of alternative systems such as the Moon.

2. **Fluctuating motivation**
    - **Frustration with slow progress**: Learning can be perceived as long and difficult.
    - **Solution**: Set realistic goals, vary teaching activities, provide psychological support.

3. **Resource accessibility**
    - **Limited availability of documents in Braille**: Not all works are available in Braille, which can limit practice.
    - **Solution**: Use connected Braille displays to access digital content, explore specialized libraries.

4. **Equipment costs**
    - **High cost of electronic devices**: Braille displays and other technologies can be expensive.
    - **Solution**: Seek financial assistance, grants or equipment loan programs.

The advantages of mastering several communication systems

1. **Flexibility and adaptability**
   Mastery of different systems enables patients to choose the most appropriate means for each situation, whether for reading, interpersonal communication or accessing information.

2. **Improved social integration**
   By using various means of communication, patients can

interact more easily with those around them, take part in social activities and access up-to-date information.

3. **Increased independence**
   The combination of Braille, voice-assist technologies and other systems expands the patient's scope for action, reducing his or her dependence on others.

Training for professional activities

Vocational training is crucial for blind people, as it promotes their independence, social inclusion and personal fulfillment. By acquiring vocational skills, blind people can gain access to rewarding jobs, actively participate in the economic and cultural life of society, and thus improve their quality of life. This approach also helps to change perceptions and combat stereotypes associated with blindness.

The importance of vocational training for blind people

Vocational training offers blind people the opportunity to develop specific skills, adapted to their abilities and aspirations. It enables them to :

- **Reinforcing autonomy**: By learning a trade, blind people gain financial independence and reduce their dependence on others.

- **Promoting social integration**: Work is a vehicle for integration, facilitating social interaction and community involvement.

- **Enhancing skills**: Training highlights the talents and skills of blind people, demonstrating that they can make a significant contribution to society.

- **Fighting discrimination**: By taking up professional positions, blind people help to change perceptions and reduce prejudices linked to visual impairment.

Challenges in accessing vocational training

Despite legislative advances and inclusion initiatives, blind people still face a number of obstacles:

- **Accessibility barriers**: Training courses are not always adapted, with inaccessible teaching aids or unequipped premises.

- **Lack of information**: Blind people may not know what training opportunities are available to them, or how to access them.

- **Prejudice and stereotypes**: Employers and trainers may have preconceived ideas about the abilities of blind people, limiting their opportunities.

- **Insufficient support** : Lack of resources, support or funding can be a barrier to enrolment and success in training programs.

Strategies for effective vocational training

1. **Adapting teaching materials and methods**

    - **Accessible materials**: Provide documents in Braille, large print or audio format for course materials.

    - **Use of assistive technologies**: Integrate screen-reading software, Braille displays or adapted mobile applications.

- **Inclusive pedagogy**: Adapt teaching methods to encourage hands-on learning, detailed verbal explanations and interactive exercises.

2. **Individualized needs assessment**

    - **Customized training plan**: Establish a program that takes into account the skills, aspirations and specific needs of each individual.

    - **Specialized support**: Trainers or tutors who are aware of blindness and can provide appropriate support.

3. **Collaboration with specialized institutions**

    - **Training centers for the visually impaired**: Work with organizations that have the expertise and resources to train blind people.

    - **Partnerships with associations**: Working with blind people's associations to facilitate access to training and employment.

4. **Financial and logistical support**

    - **Financial aid**: Information on grants, subsidies or financing schemes available to cover training and equipment costs.

    - **Reasonable accommodations**: Implementing adaptations at training sites, such as accessible premises, workstation design or adapted schedules.

5. **Raising awareness among trainers and employers**

    - **Training the trainers**: Organize awareness-raising sessions for teachers and trainers to inform them about the needs and abilities of blind people.

- **Promoting inclusion**: Encourage employers to adopt inclusive policies and recognize the added value of blind employees.

The caregiver's role in professional training

Caregivers play an essential role in helping blind people find vocational training:

- **Encouragement and motivation**: Supporting patients in their endeavors, helping them identify their skills and interests, and motivating them to pursue their career goals.

- **Information and guidance**: Provide information on training opportunities, relevant organizations and procedures.

- **Administrative assistance**: help with registration files, financial aid applications and administrative procedures.

- **Coordination with professionals**: Collaborate with trainers, guidance counselors and job placement services to ensure consistent follow-up.

- **Logistical support**: Facilitating access to training sites, helping to organize travel, or set up the necessary adaptations.

Examples of training and jobs available

Blind people can excel in many areas, depending on their skills and interests:

- **IT**: Programming, database management, technical support.

- **Human and social relations**: social work, human resources, mediation.

- **Arts and culture**: music, literature, theater, artistic creation.

- **Massage therapy and well-being**: Therapeutic massages, reflexology.

- **Administration and management**: secretarial work, accounting, project management.

- **Education and training**: Special education, Braille training, blindness awareness.

Success stories and positive impact

Many examples illustrate the success of blind people in the professional world:

- **Jacques, computer scientist**: After training in adapted programming, Jacques joined a technology company where he develops accessible applications.

- **Marie, masseuse-kinésithérapeute**: Thanks to her specialized training, Marie has opened her own massage therapy practice, where she puts her refined sense of touch to good use.

- **Ali, Braille teacher**: Ali passes on his knowledge to other blind people, contributing to their autonomy and education.

These inspiring stories show that, with the right support and resources, blind people can achieve great things.

The importance of social inclusion and combating prejudice

For vocational training for blind people to be fully effective, it is essential to create a favourable environment:

- **Raising public awareness**: Informing society about the abilities and contributions of blind people to reduce stereotypes.

- **Promoting equal opportunities**: Ensuring that public policies guarantee equitable access to training and employment.

- **Employers' commitment**: Encourage companies to recruit blind people and value diversity within their teams.

- **Ongoing support**: Follow-up after training to facilitate professional integration and job retention.

Chapter 7

Legal aspects and available resources

Rights of blind people

Blind people, like all individuals, have fundamental rights that must be recognized, respected and protected. These rights are essential to guarantee their dignity, autonomy and full participation in society. Despite the progress made, blind people continue to face obstacles that prevent them from exercising their rights. It is therefore crucial to understand these rights, the legal frameworks that support them, and the actions needed to promote and defend them.

International legal framework

At the international level, several legal instruments protect the rights of people with disabilities, including blind people:

1. **The Universal Declaration of Human Rights (1948)**: It proclaims that all human beings are born free and equal in dignity and rights, without distinction of any kind.

2. **The United Nations Convention on the Rights of Persons with Disabilities (CRPD) (2006)**: This is the first legally binding international treaty to specify the rights of people with disabilities. It aims to promote, protect and ensure the full enjoyment of all human rights by persons with disabilities, and to guarantee their equality before the law.

Key principles of the CRPD

The Convention highlights several fundamental principles:

- **Respect for intrinsic dignity**: Recognizing the inherent worth of each individual.

- **Individual autonomy**: including the freedom to make one's own choices.

- **Non-discrimination**: Prohibit all forms of discrimination based on disability.

- **Full and effective participation and inclusion in society**: Ensuring that people with disabilities can participate fully in all aspects of life.

- **Equal opportunities**: Ensuring that people with disabilities have the same opportunities as everyone else.

- **Accessibility**: Eliminating environmental, informational and communication barriers.

Specific rights of blind people

1. **The right to education**
   Blind people have the right to inclusive, quality education at all levels. This implies:

   - **Accessible teaching materials**: Use of adapted Braille, audio or digital materials.

   - **Teacher training**: Awareness-raising and training in the specific needs of blind students.

   - **Exam accommodation**: Reasonable accommodation to enable fair assessment.

2. **The right to work**
   The right to work includes access to employment and fair working conditions:

   - **Non-discrimination in hiring**: no refusal of employment on the grounds of visual disability.

   - **Reasonable accommodation**: Adaptation of workstation, tools and environment.

- **Vocational training**: Access to adapted training programs.

3. **The right to accessibility**
   Accessibility is essential for autonomy:

   - **Physical environment**: Adapting buildings, transport systems and public spaces with tactile and acoustic cues, etc.

   - **Information and communication**: Accessibility of websites and administrative documents in adapted formats.

   - **Information and communication technologies**: Development and dissemination of assistive technologies.

4. **The right to participate in cultural, recreational and sporting life**
   Blind people have the right to participate fully in cultural life:

   - **Accessibility of cultural venues**: Museums, theaters, cinemas with audiodescription systems.

   - **Sports activities**: Access to adapted sports and inclusion in general sports activities.

   - **Promoting accessible culture**: Support for literary, musical and artistic works in accessible formats.

5. **Right to privacy and autonomy**
   Respect for privacy and confidentiality :

   - **Protection of personal data**: Ensuring that personal information is treated confidentially.

- **Autonomy in decision-making**: Support for independent decision-making, including healthcare.

6. **Right to health**
   Access to health services without discrimination :

   - **Accessible health services**: Health information in adapted formats.

   - **Training medical staff**: Raising awareness of the specific needs of blind people.

7. **The right to justice**
   Equal access to justice :

   - **Adaptation of legal procedures**: legal documents in accessible formats, appropriate assistance during proceedings.

   - **Training for legal professionals**: Understanding the needs of blind people.

Implementing rights: States' responsibilities

States Parties to the CRPD are obliged to :

- **Adopt national legislation**: Incorporate the provisions of the Convention into national laws.

- **Eliminate discrimination**: Implement policies to combat discrimination and promote equality.

- **Ensure accessibility**: Develop standards and guidelines for universal accessibility.

- **Promote awareness**: Educate the public about the rights and abilities of blind people.

- **Collect data**: Gather statistics to assess policy effectiveness and identify needs.

The role of organizations of blind people

Associations and organizations play a key role:

- **Advocacy**: defending the rights and interests of blind people with governments and institutions.

- **Support and services**: Offer training, coaching and support programs.

- **Raising awareness**: Organize campaigns to change perceptions and eliminate stereotypes.

- **Policy participation**: Contribute to the development of public policy by providing real-life expertise.

Persistent challenges and the need for action

Despite legal frameworks, challenges remain:

1. **Widespread lack of accessibility**

    - **Actions required**: Investment in accessible infrastructures, technologies and services.

2. **Discrimination and stereotypes**

    - **Actions needed**: Awareness campaigns, inclusive education from an early age.

3. **High unemployment**

    - **Actions required**: Supported employment programs, incentives for employers, appropriate vocational training.

4. **Inequalities in education**

    ◦ **Action required**: Sufficient resources for inclusive schools, teacher training, accessible teaching materials.

5. **Limited access to health care**

    ◦ **Actions required**: Training of medical staff, adaptation of health services, accessible information.

Technology and innovation

Technological advances offer opportunities to improve accessibility:

- **Mobile applications**: mobility aids, object recognition, text reading.

- **Artificial intelligence**: development of tools for accessible information and communication.

- **Wearable devices**: smart glasses, connected watches with adapted functionalities.

Support organizations and associations

Support organizations and associations play a fundamental role in accompanying blind people. They are an essential pillar in fostering autonomy, social inclusion and access to education, employment and culture. These structures, often run by committed professionals and dedicated volunteers, offer a multitude of services and resources that meet the specific needs of the visually impaired. As a caregiver, it's important to be familiar with these organizations to effectively direct patients to the right resources, and thus help improve their quality of life.

The role of support organizations and associations

1. **Individual and family support**

   The associations offer personalized support to blind people and their families. They offer :

   - **Advice and guidance**: information on rights, available assistance, administrative procedures and local resources.
   - **Psychological support**: discussion groups, self-expression workshops, individual consultations to help overcome the emotional challenges of blindness.
   - **Training and education**: Braille courses, assistive technology training, vision rehabilitation programs.

2. **Promoting autonomy and social inclusion**

   - **Cultural and sporting activities**: Organization of events, cultural outings and sports clubs adapted to encourage social participation.
   - **Professional integration programs**: training workshops, internships, job coaching to help people enter the world of work.
   - **Raising public awareness**: Information campaigns to combat prejudice and promote an inclusive society.

3. **Advocacy**

   - **Representation to government bodies**: Participation in the development of public policies, advocacy for the improvement of laws and regulations in favor of blind people.

- Legal protection: Assistance in the event of discrimination, defense of individual and collective rights.
- Promoting accessibility: Actions to make public spaces, transport, information and communication accessible to all.

4. Research and innovation

    - Support for medical research: Funding of projects aimed at preventing or curing eye diseases.
    - Technological development: working with companies to create innovative tools and applications to make daily life easier for blind people.
    - Knowledge sharing: Organization of conferences, publication of guides and specialized magazines.

Main organizations and associations in France

1. **Association Valentin Haüy (AVH)**
   Founded in 1889, the AVH's mission is to help blind and partially-sighted people become more independent and fully integrated into society. Its actions include :

    - Training and employment: vocational training centers, job placement support.
    - Accessible library: Braille, audio and digital books.
    - Adapted technologies: advice on technical aids, training in their use.
    - Leisure and culture: organization of cultural, sports and leisure activities.

2. **French Federation of the Blind**
Since 1917, this federation has been working to defend the rights of visually impaired people. Its main actions are :

- **Advocacy**: Representation to public authorities, fight against discrimination.
- **Accessibility**: Promoting universal accessibility, particularly in transport and information technology.
- **Support for local associations**: Coordination and support for affiliated associations across the country.

3. **Groupement des Intellectuels Aveugles ou Amblyopes (GIAA)**
The GIAA aims to facilitate access to education, culture and information for blind and partially-sighted people. Its activities include :

- **Adaptive publishing** : Publication of magazines, books and teaching aids in accessible formats.
- **School and university support**: help with further studies, provision of adapted documents.
- **Professional integration**: support in finding skilled employment, career guidance.

4. **Association Voir Ensemble**
Created in 1927, this association offers :

- **Social and medico-social support**: reception centers, home help services.
- **Vocational training**: sheltered workshops, rehabilitation centers.
- **Leisure activities**: vacation stays, cultural and spiritual activities.

5. **Guide dogs for the blind**
Several regional associations train and provide guide dogs free of charge to blind people, improving their mobility and independence. They also offer :

- **Mobility training**: Learning how to move around with a guide dog.
- **Personalized follow-up**: Support throughout the dog's life.

How caregivers can work with these organizations

1. **Patient information and referral**

    - **Knowledge of resources**: Keep abreast of local and national associations, their services and access conditions.
    - **Appropriate referral**: Offer patients the right contacts for their specific needs.

2. **Care and service coordination**

    - **Interprofessional collaboration**: Working with professionals from associations to ensure comprehensive care.
    - **Participation in follow-up meetings**: Contribute to personalized support plans.

3. **Support with administrative formalities**

    - **Help in compiling files**: for access to services, financial aid or training offered by associations.
    - **Accompaniment to appointments**: Facilitate meetings between patient and organization representatives.

4. **Promoting autonomy**

    - **Encouraging participation**: Motivating patients to get involved in proposed activities, join support groups or workshops.
    - **Valuing skills**: Recognizing patients' talents and interests, and guiding them towards suitable programs.

The positive impact of support organizations and associations

Associations make an invaluable contribution to the lives of blind people:

- **Support networks**: They break down isolation by creating supportive communities where people can share experiences and help each other.
- **Personal development**: Through training, cultural activities and sports, they promote self-fulfilment and self-confidence.
- **Societal advances**: Their collective action helps to change attitudes, promote accessibility and defend the rights of blind people.

How to support organizations and associations

1. **Volunteer work**

    - **Participation in activities**: Offer your time to accompany outings, run workshops or support awareness-raising initiatives.
    - **Professional skills**: Provide specific skills (IT, communication, project management).

2. **Donations and funding**

    - **Financial donations**: Contribute to the financing of programs and services.

- **Fundraising**: Organize or participate in charity events.

3. **Awareness**

    - **Disseminating information**: making associations, their missions and their needs known to the general public.
    - **Promoting inclusion**: upholding the values of equality and respect in our professional and personal environment.

Access to technology and financial aid

Technology plays a crucial role in the lives of blind and partially-sighted people, providing them with tools to overcome the obstacles associated with vision loss. These assistive technologies improve autonomy, facilitate communication, access to information, mobility and social integration. However, the high cost of these devices can be a major barrier for many people. That's why it's essential to be aware of the various financial aids available to facilitate access to these technologies. As a caregiver, your role is to support patients in obtaining these resources, informing them of the options available and accompanying them through the administrative process.

The importance of assistive technologies for blind people

Assistive technologies are devices or software designed to compensate for the functional limitations associated with a disability. For blind people, they enable :

- **Communicate effectively**: Screen readers, voice synthesizers and electronic Braille devices provide access to computers, smartphones and the Internet.
- **Accessing information**: Mobile applications and OCR (optical character recognition) scanners transform printed text into audio, making documents, books and newspapers easier to read.
- **Getting around safely**: adapted GPS, electronic walking sticks and assisted navigation applications improve mobility and orientation.
- **Managing everyday tasks**: Voice-controlled home automation devices can manage lighting, heating and household appliances.
- **Participating in social and professional life**: Technologies facilitate access to education, vocational training and employment.

The different types of assistive technology

1. **Screen readers and voice synthesizers**: convert text displayed on a screen into voice synthesis. Examples: JAWS, NVDA, VoiceOver (for Apple devices).

2. **Electronic Braille displays**: These devices display the text content of a computer or smartphone in Braille, enabling tactile reading.

3. **Optical character recognition (OCR) software**: transforms printed documents into digital text that can be read by voice synthesis or Braille.

4. **Specific mobile applications**: Object, color and banknote recognition applications such as Seeing AI, Be My Eyes or TapTapSee.

5. **Mobility devices**: electronic white cane, adapted GPS, haptic feedback guidance devices.

6. **Accessible home automation**: Voice commands to control home appliances, such as voice assistants (Amazon Alexa, Google Assistant).

The costs associated with assistive technologies

Despite their usefulness, these technologies often represent a significant financial investment. Specialized devices, such as electronic Braille displays or professional software, can cost several thousand euros. Costs can include :

- **Purchase of the device**: High cost of specialized equipment.
- **Software**: Some screen-reading software is not free.
- **Training**: Learning how to use technology.
- **Maintenance and updates**: Costs associated with technical support and software updates.

Financial assistance available

To overcome these financial obstacles, a number of grants and subsidies are available in France:

1. **The Disability Compensation Scheme (PCH)**

    - **Description**: The PCH is a financial aid designed to cover disability-related expenses, including the acquisition of technical aids.
    - **Eligibility requirements**: Recognized disability, stable and regular residence in France, and absolute difficulty in performing an essential activity or serious difficulty in at least two activities.
    - **Steps**: Apply to the Maison Départementale des Personnes Handicapées (MDPH), with a file including a medical certificate, a life project and an assessment of needs.

2. **Disabled Adult Allowance (AAH)**

    - **Description**: The AAH guarantees a minimum income for people with disabilities.
    - **Use**: Although intended to provide income, it can indirectly contribute to the financing of assistive technologies.
    - **Eligibility requirements**: disability recognized by the MDPH, income below a certain ceiling.

3. **AGEFIPH and FIPHFP grants**

    - **AGEFIPH** (Association de Gestion du Fonds pour l'Insertion Professionnelle des Personnes Handicapées) for the private sector.
    - **FIPHFP** (Fonds pour l'Insertion des Personnes Handicapées dans la Fonction Publique) for the public sector.
    - **Description**: These organizations finance technical aids to promote professional integration.
    - **Utilization**: Financing of adapted equipment, adaptation of workstations.
    - **Procedures**: Through your employer or human resources department.

4. **Assistance from mutual insurers and insurance companies**

    - **Description**: Some supplementary health insurance plans provide reimbursements for the purchase of technical aids.
    - **Steps to take**: Check the clauses of your insurance or mutual insurance contract, and contact your advisor for details.

5. **Subsidies from associations and foundations**

    - **Examples**: Association Valentin Haüy, Fédération des Aveugles de France, Fondation ONCE.
    - **Description**: These organizations offer financial assistance, equipment loans or partial financing.
    - **Procedure**: Contact the associations directly to find out about available programs.

6. **Local assistance**

    - **Description**: Some local authorities (communes, départements, regions) offer specific assistance.
    - **Procedure**: Contact your local social services or Centre Communal d'Action Sociale (CCAS).

7. **Tax credits and deductions**

    - **Description**: Expenditure on home improvements and equipment may be eligible for tax benefits.
    - **Steps to take**: Consult a tax adviser or the tax authorities to find out about the schemes in force.

The caregiver's role in accessing technology and financial aid

As a caregiver, you can play a key role in facilitating patient access to assistive technologies:

1. **Information and awareness-raising**

    - **Knowledge of resources**: Keep abreast of available technologies and financial assistance.
    - **Patient communication**: Explain the benefits of assistive technologies and how they can improve quality of life.

2. **Administrative support**

    ○ **Helping to compile files**: Supporting the patient in collecting the necessary documents, drafting requests and meeting deadlines.
    ○ **Referral to appropriate services**: Put patients in touch with social workers, associations or administrative services.

3. **Training and support for technology use**

    ○ **Facilitate learning**: help patients familiarize themselves with new devices, organize training sessions.
    ○ **Follow-up and encouragement**: Encourage regular use of technology, answer questions and resolve any problems.

4. **Coordination with healthcare professionals and specialists**

    ○ **Interprofessional collaboration**: Work with occupational therapists, orthoptists and locomotion instructors, for a holistic approach.
    ○ **Sharing information**: Transmit observations on patient needs, difficulties encountered and progress made.

5. **Promoting autonomy**

    ○ **Confidence-building**: Valuing the patient's efforts, highlighting the concrete benefits of technology on his or her autonomy.
    ○ **Patient involvement**: Encourage patients to express their preferences and actively participate in equipment selection.

Steps to obtain financial aid

1. **Needs assessment**

    - **Functional assessment**: work with professionals to assess the need for technical aids.
    - **Medical prescription**: Obtain a prescription or detailed prescription for the devices required.

2. **Information search**

    - **Identifying available assistance**: List the financial mechanisms adapted to the patient's situation.
    - **Document collection** : Gather the required supporting documents (medical certificates, proof of income, etc.).

3. **File creation and submission**

    - **Writing requests**: Fill in forms accurately, clearly describing your needs.
    - **Submitting files**: Respect procedures and deadlines.

4. **Request follow-up**

    - **Follow-up if necessary**: Contact organizations to ensure that files are received and processed correctly.
    - **Response to additional requests**: Provide additional information if requested.

5. **Use of grants**

    - **Purchasing equipment**: Purchase equipment in compliance with the terms and conditions of the grants (quotes or invoices are sometimes required).

- ◦ **Justification of expenses**: Keep proof of purchase for possible audits.

Potential obstacles and how to overcome them

- **Administrative complexity**: The process can be long and complex. **Solution**: Get help from a professional or an association.

- **Processing times** : Processing times can be long. **Solution**: Anticipate requests and provide temporary solutions if necessary.

- **Refusal of assistance**: Requests may be refused. **Solution**: Understand the reasons for the refusal, lodge an appeal if possible, or look for alternatives.

Additional resources

- **Technical aids information and advice centers (CICAT)**: provide information on available equipment.

- **Maisons Départementales des Personnes Handicapées (MDPH)**: the central point for disability-related procedures.

- **Social workers**: can help you navigate the system of benefits and assistance.

- **Specialized websites**: offer up-to-date information on financial aids and technologies (for example, the CNSA or Ministry of Solidarity and Health websites).

Chapter 8

Technological innovations in the care of the blind

Modern devices and assistive technologies

- **Mobility aids**
  - Electronic rods

Electronic rods

Mobility is fundamental to the autonomy and quality of life of blind and partially-sighted people. The white cane is one of the essential tools for mobility. However, with technological advances, the traditional white cane has evolved to incorporate electronic devices, giving rise to electronic canes. These innovative tools offer additional functionalities that enhance obstacle detection and safety when on the move. Understanding how electronic canes work, their benefits, and the associated challenges, is crucial for healthcare professionals, patients and their families.

From the white cane to the electronic cane

The white cane was introduced at the beginning of the XXe century as a symbol of blindness and a practical tool for detecting obstacles on the ground. It enables users to feel variations in the terrain, locate steps, kerbs and objects on the ground. However, it does have its limitations, particularly in detecting overhead obstacles such as tree branches, signs or protruding parts of buildings.

To overcome these limitations, engineers and researchers have developed electronic canes, which incorporate sensors and advanced technologies to improve obstacle detection, not only on the ground, but also at head and torso level. These devices aim to increase the safety, efficiency and confidence of blind people as they move around.

How electronic rods work

Electronic canes are traditional white canes to which electronic components have been added. They are equipped with sensors, usually ultrasonic, infrared or laser, which detect obstacles in the user's immediate environment. When the cane detects an obstacle, it warns the user by means of tactile signals (vibrations), auditory signals (beeps) or sometimes by vocal indications.

Here's how an electronic rod generally works:

1. **Obstacle detection**: sensors emit waves (ultrasound, infrared) which reflect off surrounding objects. The device measures the return time of the waves to calculate the distance between the user and the obstacle.

2. **Alerting the user**: Depending on the distance of the obstacle, the cane emits alerts in the form of vibrations of varying intensity or sounds of varying frequency. This enables the user to assess the proximity and nature of the obstacle.

3. **Sensor range**: The effective range of the sensors generally varies between one and four meters, giving you plenty of room to react and adjust your trajectory.

4. **Power supply**: Electronic rods run on rechargeable batteries. Autonomy varies according to model and use.

Advantages of electronic rods

Electronic rods offer several significant advantages over traditional white rods:

- **High obstacle detection**: These detect obstacles above cane level, avoiding collisions with objects that the white cane cannot detect.

- **Increased safety**: By providing additional information on the environment, they reduce the risk of accidents and increase user confidence.

- **Improved mobility**: users can move around faster and with greater ease, knowing that they have advance warning of obstacles.

- **Personalized alerts** : Some models allow you to adjust the intensity of vibrations or the volume of sounds, according to the user's preferences.

- **Integration of additional functions**: Some devices integrate functions such as electronic compass, GPS and smartphone connectivity, offering advanced navigation and orientation services.

Examples of electronic rods

Several models of electronic rods are available on the market, each offering specific features:

- **TOM POUCE electronic cane**: Developed in France, this cane is equipped with ultrasonic sensors that detect obstacles at head height. It alerts the user by vibrating the handle.

- **The UltraCane electronic cane**: Originating in the UK, it uses ultrasonic sensors to detect obstacles at the front and at height. Signals are transmitted via separate vibrations for each sensor, making it possible to distinguish the position of obstacles.

- **The WeWALK cane**: This is a smart cane that integrates sensors, Bluetooth connectivity and navigation functions. It connects to a smartphone to offer voice directions, route recognition and integration with applications such as Google Maps.

- **RAY electronic walking stick**: combines obstacle detection with GPS and communication functions. It can provide voice guidance on the environment and directions to follow.

Limitations and challenges of electronic rods

Despite their advantages, electronic rods have certain limitations:

- **Complexity of use**: Learning to use an electronic cane can be more complex than learning to use a traditional white cane. It requires specific training to interpret signals correctly and react accordingly.

- **Sensor reliability**: Sensor performance can be affected by environmental conditions such as rain, fog or wave-absorbing obstacles, which can reduce their effectiveness.

- **Weight and ergonomics**: Electronic components add weight to the rod, which can make handling more tiring. Balance and ergonomics must be carefully considered.

- **High cost**: Electronic rods are generally more expensive than traditional white rods, which can be a financial obstacle for some users.

- **Energy dependency**: Operation depends on the power supply. A battery failure can leave the user without electronic functionality, or even without a cane if it is not designed for passive operation.

The role of the caregiver in supporting the use of electronic canes

As a caregiver, you have a crucial role to play in supporting patients who wish to use an electronic cane:

- **Information and awareness**: Present the various electronic cane options, explain how they work and their benefits, and help patients determine whether this tool is right for them.

- **Referral**: Connect the patient with specialized locomotion instructors, who are trained to teach the use of electronic walking sticks.

- **Support during training**: Accompany the patient during training sessions, provide moral support, and help repeat exercises if necessary.

- **Assistance with administrative formalities**: Helping patients to obtain the financial aid available for the purchase of an electronic cane, by assisting them in the preparation of applications to the relevant organizations.

- **Follow-up and encouragement**: After acquiring the cane, monitor the patient's progress, encourage him/her to use the device regularly, and be alert to any difficulties encountered and report them to the relevant professionals.

Financial aid for the acquisition of an electronic walking stick

The high cost of electronic canes can be partially or fully covered by various financial aid schemes:

- **Prestation de Compensation du Handicap (PCH)**: This can cover the cost of technical aids, including electronic walking sticks.

- **Mutuelles and insurance companies**: Some complementary health insurance companies offer fixed-price packages for medical equipment.

- **Associations**: Organizations such as the Association Valentin Haüy or the Fédération des Aveugles de France can provide financial assistance or facilitate access to loan schemes.

- **Local subsidies**: Some local authorities offer grants for the purchase of equipment for disabled people.

Choosing the right electronic cane

When choosing an electronic cane, several criteria must be taken into account:

- **The patient's specific needs**: level of visual impairment, physical capabilities, travel environment (urban, rural).

- **Ease of use**: simple controls, signal interpretation, ergonomics.

- **Features offered**: Sensor range, alert types, integration with mobile devices, additional features (GPS, compass).

- **Reliability and robustness**: build quality, weather resistance, battery life.

- **Available budget**: cost of equipment, financing options.

We recommend trying out several models, if possible, and consulting professionals for expert advice.

Training in the use of the electronic cane

Mastering the electronic cane requires training by instructors specializing in locomotion:

- **Learn basic techniques**: cane handling, sweeping techniques, obstacle detection.

- **Interpreting signals**: Understand vibrations or sounds emitted by the cane, associate these signals with surrounding obstacles.

- **Adaptability to a variety of environments**: practice indoors and outdoors, in calm and then more complex environments.

- **Handling special situations**: stairs, narrow passages, street crossings, moving obstacles.

Training is essential to ensure user safety and take full advantage of the electronic rod's functionalities.

Maintenance and care of electronic rods

To ensure proper operation of the electronic cane, it is important to :

- **Regular maintenance**: clean sensors, check general condition, check for damage.

- **Check power supply**: recharge batteries according to manufacturer's recommendations, carry spare batteries if necessary.

- **Software updates**: For connected rods, perform software updates to benefit from improvements and corrections.

- **Consult the after-sales service**: In case of malfunction, contact the manufacturer or dealer for technical assistance.

Future prospects for electronic rods

Research and development in the field of assistive technology for blind people is constantly evolving. Electronic canes continue to improve thanks to technological advances:

- **Integration of artificial intelligence**: for more precise obstacle recognition, object classification and contextual guidance.

- **Improved ergonomics**: reduced weight, more compact design, more resistant materials.

- **Increased connectivity**: Interaction with mobile devices, access to real-time information, integration with navigation services.

- **Affordability**: Development of more affordable models to democratize access to these technologies.

○ Customized GPS navigation systems

Customized GPS navigation systems

Autonomous mobility is an essential element in the independence and quality of life of blind and partially sighted people. Travelling in unfamiliar or complex environments can represent a considerable challenge due to the absence of visual cues. Adapted GPS navigation systems have emerged as valuable tools for overcoming these obstacles, providing real-time information on the environment and guiding users safely to their destination. These innovative technologies combine advances in global positioning with user interfaces specially designed to meet the needs of the visually impaired.

The importance of GPS navigation systems for blind people

GPS (Global Positioning System) navigation systems have revolutionized the way people get around, offering precise location and route guidance. For blind people, these adapted systems are much more than just a comfort tool; they represent an opportunity to broaden their range of mobility, reduce dependence on others and increase their confidence when traveling. By providing detailed information on the environment, adapted GPS systems help to :

- **Identify streets, intersections and landmarks**: Understand the layout of the surrounding area.
- **Plan optimal routes**: Choose the safest, most direct route to a destination.
- **Receive real-time alerts**: Be informed of route changes, roadworks or temporary obstacles.
- **Facilitate exploration of new places**: Encourage autonomy in unfamiliar environments.

Characteristics of suitable GPS navigation systems

GPS systems for blind people incorporate specific functionalities to compensate for the absence of vision and make the most of the other senses, in particular hearing and touch. Here are the main features of these systems:

1. **Voice guidance**

    - **Detailed audio instructions**: Navigation instructions are provided in the form of clear, precise voice messages, including distance to next turning point, street names, nearby points of interest.
    - **Voice customization**: Choose your voice synthesis timbre, speed and language for optimum comfort.

2. **Touch and haptic interface**

    - **Vibratory feedback**: Devices can emit specific vibrations to signal actions or alerts, useful in noisy environments.
    - **Adapted touch screens**: Smartphone applications incorporate simplified gestures and

enlarged touch zones to facilitate interaction without looking at the screen.

3. **Integration with assistive devices**

   ◦ **Screen reader compatibility**: GPS applications are designed to work with screen readers such as VoiceOver (iOS) or TalkBack (Android).
   ◦ **Connection with electronic rods or connected watches**: For a seamless, integrated navigation experience.

4. **Enriched environmental information**

   ◦ **Intersection description**: type of intersection (crossroads, traffic circle), number of lanes to be crossed.
   ◦ **Points of interest**: Information on public buildings, bus stops and shops, with useful descriptions for the user.
   ◦ **Obstacle alerts**: warn of work zones, inaccessible sidewalks or potential hazards.

5. **Advanced orientation features**

   ◦ **Indoor navigation**: Some applications offer guidance services in public buildings, railway stations and shopping malls, using Bluetooth or Wi-Fi technology.
   ◦ **Optimized pedestrian mode**: Routes are adapted to pedestrians, with priority given to safe sidewalks and crosswalks.

6. **Personalization and learning**

   ◦ **Favorites and personalized itineraries**: Frequent destinations can be saved for quick access.

- **Machine learning**: systems can adapt to user preferences by learning from their travel habits.

Examples of suitable GPS navigation systems

Several applications and devices have been developed specifically for blind people:

1. **BlindSquare**

    - **Description**: iOS application that uses Foursquare and OpenStreetMap data to provide environmental information.
    - **Features**: Announce intersections, nearby points of interest, set destinations and receive detailed instructions.

2. **Lazarillo**

    - **Description**: Available on iOS and Android, Lazarillo offers real-time voice guidance.
    - **Features**: information on streets, shops and public transport stops, with an interface compatible with screen readers.

3. **Google Maps with improved accessibility**

    - **Description**: Although not specifically designed for the blind, Google Maps has integrated accessibility features.
    - **Features**: Detailed voice instructions for pedestrian routes, alerts on crossings and changes of direction.

4. **Microsoft Soundscape**

    ○ **Description**: An application for iOS that uses 3D audio to help build a mental image of the environment.
    ○ **Features**: Spatialized sound emissions to indicate the direction of points of interest, possibility of defining personal audio beacons.

5. **Kapten Mobility**

    ○ **Description**: A GPS navigation assistant dedicated to blind people, available in France.
    ○ **Features**: precise voice guidance, environmental information, easy-to-use interface.

Challenges and limitations of adapted GPS systems

Despite their many advantages, these systems have certain limitations:

- **GPS signal accuracy**: In dense urban environments or indoors, GPS accuracy may be reduced, affecting the reliability of indications.
- **Connectivity dependency**: Many applications require an Internet connection to access map data and real-time information.
- **Interface complexity**: Some users may encounter difficulties with application interfaces, requiring training or support.
- **Data updates**: Information on infrastructure and points of interest must be regularly updated to remain relevant.
- **Cost**: While some applications are free, others may require purchase or subscription, and the use of mobile data may incur additional costs.

The role of the caregiver in supporting the use of adapted GPS systems

As a caregiver, you play a key role in helping patients take full advantage of adapted GPS navigation systems:

1. **Information and awareness-raising**
    - **Present available options**: Inform patients about the different applications and devices available, taking into account their needs and preferences.
    - **Explain the benefits**: Emphasize how these technologies can improve autonomy and safety on the move.

2. **Installation and configuration support**
    - **Technical assistance**: Assist the patient in downloading, installing and initially configuring the application or device.
    - **Customize settings**: Adjust settings (voice, volume, language) for an optimal experience.

3. **User training**
    - **Hands-on sessions**: Organize sessions to familiarize the patient with the necessary functions, commands and interactions.
    - **Real-life scenarios**: Accompany the patient on real-life journeys to practice using the system under authentic conditions.

4. **Ongoing support**
    - **Problem solving**: Helping to overcome technical or user difficulties that may arise.
    - **Updating knowledge**: Inform patients of new features or important updates.

5. **Coordination with specialized professionals**

    ◦ **Collaboration with locomotion instructors**: Work in synergy with professionals who teach locomotion techniques to effectively integrate the use of GPS systems.

Financial aid for the acquisition of adapted GPS devices

Access to adapted technologies can be facilitated by various forms of financial aid:

- **Prestation de Compensation du Handicap (PCH)**: Can cover part of the cost of acquiring technical aids.
- **Associations and foundations**: Some organizations offer financing, loans or equipment donations.
- **Mutuelles and insurance**: Check with your complementary health insurance provider to find out what coverage is available.
- **Local subsidies**: Local authorities can offer subsidies for the purchase of assistive technology.

Technological advances and the future of navigation systems for blind people

The field of assistive technologies is constantly evolving, paving the way for significant improvements:

- **Artificial Intelligence (AI)**: AI enables more precise recognition of the environment, real-time obstacle detection and more contextual guidance.
- **Augmented Reality (AR)**: Integration of AR to provide enriched information about the environment via audio or tactile devices.
- **Collaborative cartography**: users can contribute to the enrichment of cartographic data, improving the accuracy and relevance of information.

- **Haptic technologies**: Development of devices offering more sophisticated tactile feedback, such as vibrating wristbands or connected shoes.

- **Voice and visual recognition technologies**
  - Screen reader applications

Screen reader applications

Access to information and communication is essential for the autonomy and social integration of people who are blind or partially sighted. Screen-reading applications play a crucial role in enabling these people to use computers, smartphones and other digital devices. They transform the visual content displayed on the screen into audible or Braille information, opening up a world of possibilities for education, work, leisure and communication. As a caregiver, it's important to understand how these applications work, their benefits and limitations, and how you can support patients in their use.

What is a screen reader application?

A screen reader application is software that interprets the textual and graphical content of a computer, smartphone or tablet screen, and converts it into text-to-speech or Braille via a Braille display. It enables blind or partially-sighted users to navigate interfaces, access information, enter text and interact with applications, replacing or supplementing visual perception with auditory or tactile means.

How screen reader applications work

Screen reader applications work by interacting with the operating system and applications to extract information displayed on the screen. Here's how they work:

1. **Content interpretation**: The screen reader analyzes the structure of the user interface, including text, images, menus, buttons and input fields.

2. **Focus management**: tracks the user's focus, i.e. the element they are currently on, and provides contextual information about this element.

3. **Text-to-speech**: Text is converted into synthetic speech using a text-to-speech engine, with the option of choosing voice, speed and language.

4. **Braille display**: For users with a Braille display, the screen reader sends the text to the device, which translates it into tactile Braille characters.

5. **Specific commands**: Users can interact with the screen reader using keyboard shortcuts, touch gestures or voice commands to navigate, read and control the interface.

Main screen reader applications

There are several screen-reading applications, some of which are integrated into operating systems, others available as third-party software:

1. **NVDA (NonVisual Desktop Access)**
    - **Platform** : Windows
    - **Description**: NVDA is a free, open-source screen reader that offers an affordable alternative to paid software. It supports numerous applications and web browsers, and is compatible with Braille displays.
    - **Features**: Multilingual speech synthesis, Office application support, efficient web browsing, regular updates.

2. **JAWS (Job Access With Speech)**
    - **Platform** : Windows
    - **Description**: JAWS is one of the most popular and powerful screen readers, but it has to be paid for. It offers a wide range of advanced features for professional use.
    - **Features**: Extensive application support, advanced customization, specific scripts for complex applications, integration with Braille displays.

3. **VoiceOver**
    - **Platform**: macOS, iOS (iPhone, iPad)
    - **Description**: VoiceOver is integrated into Apple devices, delivering a smooth, consistent experience on Mac computers, iPhones and iPads.
    - **Features**: iOS gesture controls, deep system integration, native app support, high-quality voice.

4. **TalkBack**
    - **Platform** : Android
    - **Description**: TalkBack is the screen reader provided by Google for Android devices. It lets users interact with their smartphones and tablets using touch gestures.
    - **Features**: Gesture navigation, multilingual support, customizable preferences, integration with Google applications.

5. **Narrator**
    - **Platform** : Windows

- **Description**: Narrator is Windows' built-in screen reader. It has been enhanced in recent versions to offer a more complete experience.
- **Features**: Easy access, no installation required, basic support for common applications.

6. **SuperNova**

    - **Platform** : Windows
    - **Description**: SuperNova offers both screen-reading and magnification functions for the visually impaired.
    - **Features**: Voice synthesis, Braille support, screen magnification, high contrast options.

Advantages of screen reader applications

1. **Access to information**

    - **Internet browsing** : Screen readers let you browse the web, access sites, read articles and fill in online forms.
    - **Using applications**: They make office software, e-mail, social networks, etc. accessible.

2. **Autonomy in daily tasks**

    - **Email management**: Read, write and send emails.
    - **Word processing**: Create and edit documents.

3. **Participation in professional and educational life**

    - **Studies**: Access to digital teaching resources, participation in online courses.
    - **Work**: Use of professional tools, collaboration with colleagues.

4. **Communication and leisure**
    - **Social networks**: Interaction on Facebook, Twitter and other platforms.
    - **Entertainment**: Read e-books, listen to music, watch videos with audio description.

Limitations and challenges of screen-reading applications

1. **Application compatibility**
    - **Variable accessibility**: Not all applications are designed with accessibility in mind, which can make them difficult or impossible to use with a screen reader.
    - **Interface complexity**: Complex graphical interfaces or applications rich in visual content can be challenging.

2. **Learning curve**
    - **Training required**: Mastering the use of a screen reader takes time and practice, especially for those less familiar with the technology.
    - **Shortcuts and commands**: Many keyboard shortcuts and gestures need to be memorized to navigate efficiently.

3. **Performance and responsiveness**
    - **System resources**: Some screen readers can be resource-hungry, affecting computer performance.
    - **Response times**: Delays in speech synthesis can adversely affect the user experience.

4. **Costs**

   - **Paid software**: Applications like JAWS are expensive, which can be an obstacle for some users.

The role of the caregiver in supporting the use of screen-reading applications

1. **Information and awareness-raising**

   - **Present the available options**: Inform patients of the different applications, their advantages and disadvantages, taking into account their needs and level of technological expertise.
   - **Explain the benefits**: Emphasize how these tools can improve autonomy and access to information.

2. **Installation and configuration**

   - **Technical assistance**: Assist the patient with software installation, initial configuration, and adaptation of parameters (voice, reading speed, language).
   - **Personalization**: Adjust settings to suit patient preferences, such as choice of text-to-speech or commands.

3. **Training and apprenticeships**

   - **Introduction to the basics**: teach the essential commands for navigating, reading text and using common applications.
   - **Guided practice**: Organize practical sessions to reinforce skills, resolve difficulties and answer questions.

- **Educational resources**: Provide guides, tutorials, or links to appropriate online training courses.

4. **Ongoing support**

    - **Troubleshooting**: Helping to resolve technical problems, errors or software updates.
    - **Encouragement**: Motivate patients to persevere despite challenges, reward progress.

5. **Coordination with professionals**

    - **Collaboration with specialized trainers**: Put the patient in touch with instructors in adapted computing or associations offering training courses.
    - **Monitoring needs**: Adapting support to the patient's evolving skills and goals.

Financial assistance for the acquisition of screen-reading software

- **Prestation de Compensation du Handicap (PCH)**: Can cover the cost of acquiring assistive software.
- **Associations and foundations**: Some organizations offer financial assistance, discounted licenses or free training courses.
- **Corporate accessibility programs**: Some companies offer free or reduced-price licenses for people with disabilities.
- **Mutuelles and insurance**: Check with your complementary health insurance provider to find out what coverage is available.

Promoting digital accessibility

Beyond the use of screen readers, it's important to promote digital accessibility so that websites, applications and documents are designed to be inclusive. Accessibility principles include:

- **Use of semantic tags**: So that screen readers can interpret content correctly.
- **Alternative descriptions for images**: Provide descriptive text for visual elements.
- **Keyboard navigation**: Enable navigation without a mouse.
- **Appropriate color contrasts**: make reading easier for the visually impaired.

Technological advances and the future of screen-reading applications

Technological advances continue to improve screen readers:

- **Artificial Intelligence (AI)**: AI enables better content interpretation, automatic image description and character recognition in images.
- **Integration with voice assistants**: assistants like Siri, Alexa or Google Assistant offer additional ways of interacting with devices.
- **Cost reduction**: The rise of open-source software and the integration of screen readers into operating systems are reducing financial barriers.
- **Universal accessibility**: Increased awareness of accessibility is encouraging developers to design applications compatible with screen readers from the outset.

- Object and text recognition software

Object and text recognition software

Technology has evolved considerably over the last few decades, offering innovative solutions to improve the quality of life of blind and partially-sighted people. Among these advances, object and text recognition software occupy a prominent place. They enable visually impaired people to access visual information in their environment by converting it into auditory or tactile data. These revolutionary tools promote autonomy, facilitate daily activities and reinforce social inclusion. Understanding how they work, their benefits and limitations, and the role caregivers can play in their use, is essential to maximizing their positive impact.

Understanding object and text recognition software

Object and text recognition software uses artificial intelligence (AI) and computer vision to analyze images captured by a camera, usually that of a smartphone, and extract meaningful information. They can identify objects, read printed or handwritten text, recognize faces, colors, banknotes, and even describe complex scenes. This information is then returned to the user in the form of voice synthesis, vibration or Braille display.

How recognition software works

1. **Image capture**: Users point their device's camera at the object or text they wish to identify. Some software packages can also process images already stored.

2. **Image analysis**: The software uses deep learning algorithms to analyze the image. For text recognition, it uses Optical Character Recognition (OCR) to extract the text present in the image.

3. **Data interpretation** : For object recognition, the software compares image features with a database of known objects to identify what is being captured.

4. **Information feedback**: Results are communicated to the user via a voice synthesizer that describes the object or reads the text. Some programs also offer tactile feedback or specific sound notifications.

Importance for blind and partially sighted people

This software is a major asset for the visually impaired:

- **Increased autonomy**: They enable you to carry out everyday tasks without assistance, such as reading a menu in a restaurant, identifying products in the supermarket, or choosing an item of clothing.

- **Access to information**: The ability to read printed documents, notice boards or labels facilitates access to education, work and leisure.

- **Enhanced safety**: By identifying obstacles or potential hazards, these tools contribute to safety on the move.

- **Social interaction**: Facial recognition can help identify people in a group, facilitating social interaction.

Examples of software and applications

1. **Seeing AI** (Microsoft)
    - **Description**: A free application for iOS that describes the user's immediate environment.
    - **Features** :
        - Read short texts in real time.

- Document recognition with guidance for optimum capture.
- Product identification via barcode.
- Scene description and face recognition with age and emotion estimation.
- Banknote detection.

2. **Envision AI**

    - **Description** : Available on iOS and Android, Envision AI offers a full range of recognition features.

    - **Features** :

        - Reading of printed and handwritten texts in over 60 languages.
        - Description of complex scenes.
        - Identification of specific objects through personalized training.
        - Color and light recognition.

3. **KNFB Reader**

    - **Description** : A powerful text reader available on iOS and Android.

    - **Features** :

        - Fast, high-precision reading of printed documents.
        - Ability to read columnar documents, labels and computer screens.
        - Save and share scanned documents.

4. **Be My Eyes**

    ○ **Description**: An innovative application that connects blind people with sighted volunteers via a video call.

    ○ **Features** :

    - Human assistance for occasional tasks, such as reading an expiration date, checking the color of a garment, or adjusting a thermostat.

5. **Supersense**

    ○ **Description**: An Android application that uses AI to help with various tasks.

    ○ **Features** :

    - Reading texts, including handwritten ones.
    - Exploration of the environment with object identification.
    - Assistance with indoor navigation by pointing the camera at the environment.

Advantages of recognition software

- **Versatility**: a single application can offer multiple functionalities, reducing the need for several separate tools.

- **Availability**: Most of this software is available on everyday smartphones, avoiding the need to purchase expensive specialized devices.

- **Regular updates**: Developers are constantly improving algorithms, increasing accuracy and adding new features.

- **Customization**: Some programs allow you to customize settings to meet specific user needs, such as language selection, reading speed, or types of information required.

Limitations and challenges

- **Variable accuracy**: Recognition accuracy can be affected by image quality, lighting conditions or environmental complexity.

- **Connectivity dependency**: Some software requires an Internet connection to operate, which can be problematic in areas without a network.

- **Learning curve**: A certain amount of familiarization is required to use these tools effectively, particularly for framing the camera correctly.

- **Confidentiality**: Using online services raises confidentiality issues, as images may be processed on remote servers.

- **Language barrier**: Not all applications are available in all languages, or offer optimal recognition for certain languages.

The caregiver's role in supporting the use of recognition software

1. **Information and awareness-raising**

    - **Present the available options**: Inform the patient about the different applications, highlighting their features and benefits.

- **Explain the benefits**: Show how these tools can facilitate daily tasks and improve autonomy.

2. **Installation and configuration**

    - **Technical assistance**: Assist the patient in downloading, installing and initially configuring the application.
    - **Customization**: adapt settings to suit patient preferences, such as language, synthesized voice or notifications.

3. **User training**

    - **Practical demonstration**: Show how to use the application in real-life situations, such as reading a document or identifying an object.
    - **Shooting guidance**: Teach how to position the camera to optimize recognition, taking into account angle, distance and lighting.
    - **Problem-solving**: Helping to understand and overcome errors or difficulties encountered during use.

4. **Ongoing support**

    - **Encouragement**: Motivate the patient to use the applications on a regular basis to gain confidence and ease of use.
    - **Updates**: Inform about new features or improvements brought by updates.
    - **Feedback to developers**: Encourage patients to share their experiences to help improve applications.

Financial assistance for the acquisition of software and equipment

Although many applications are free or inexpensive, the purchase of a compatible smartphone or data subscription can represent a significant expense. Financial assistance is available:

- **Prestation de Compensation du Handicap (PCH)**: Can cover the cost of technical aids, including smartphones and pay-per-use applications.

- **Associations and foundations**: Some organizations offer grants or equipment on loan.

- **Mutuelles and insurance**: Check with complementary health insurance companies to find out if they will cover your costs.

- **Special programs**: Some manufacturers or telephone operators offer reduced rates for people with disabilities.

Promoting autonomy and inclusion

The use of object and text recognition software not only contributes to the autonomy of blind people, but also to their social inclusion:

- **Active participation**: By facilitating access to information, these tools enable individuals to participate fully in educational, professional and cultural activities.

- **Reduced dependency**: Less need to seek help from others for simple tasks, boosting self-confidence.

- **Raising awareness**: By demonstrating the technological capabilities available, we encourage a positive perception of the skills of blind people.

Technological advances and future prospects

The field of object and text recognition is constantly evolving, with significant improvements expected:

- **Advanced artificial intelligence**: Algorithms become more precise, capable of understanding complex contexts and providing more detailed descriptions.

- **Multimodal recognition**: Combining visual analysis with other sensors (sound, motion) for a richer understanding of the environment.

- **Offline operation**: Development of applications capable of operating without an Internet connection, thanks to the integration of AI models directly on the device.

- **Enhanced accessibility**: simplified interfaces, voice commands and integration with other assistive technologies.

- **Smart glasses and augmented reality**

Technology is evolving at a breathtaking pace, offering new opportunities to improve the quality of life of blind and partially sighted people. Among these advances, smart glasses and augmented reality take pride of place. These innovative devices combine sophisticated hardware, sensors, cameras and software to provide real-time information about the environment, transforming the way visually impaired people interact with the world around them. As a caregiver, understanding the potential of these technologies enables us to better support patients in their quest for autonomy and social inclusion.

Understanding smart glasses and augmented reality

Smart glasses are wearable devices that resemble ordinary eyewear, but incorporate advanced electronic components. Augmented reality (AR), meanwhile, is a technology that superimposes digital information on physical reality, enriching the user's perception. For the blind or visually impaired, these technologies can transform visual information into auditory or tactile signals, offering a new sensory dimension.

How smart glasses work for blind people

Smart glasses for the visually impaired use a combination of cameras, sensors and artificial intelligence software to analyze the environment. Here's how they usually work:

1. **Environmental capture**: On-board cameras capture real-time images of the user's environment.

2. **Data analysis and processing**: Artificial intelligence software processes these images to recognize objects, text, faces, obstacles and even facial expressions.

3. **Information restitution**: The analyzed information is transmitted to the user via auditory signals (headphones or bone conduction) or tactile signals (vibrations), enabling him to understand and interact with his environment.

Advantages of smart glasses and augmented reality

1. **Improved mobility and orientation**
    - **Obstacle detection**: the glasses can warn the user of obstacles in their path, improving safety while on the move.
    - **Real-time guidance**: integrated with suitable GPS systems, they can provide precise navigation indications.

2. **Access to information**

    - **Text reading**: Thanks to optical character recognition (OCR), they can read signs, menus, labels and other texts, restoring information by voice synthesis.
    - **Object recognition**: Identification of everyday objects, making tasks such as shopping or meal preparation easier.

3. **Enhanced social interaction**

    - **Facial recognition**: Identification of known people, combined with the ability to detect facial expressions, helping to interpret emotions and improve social interactions.
    - **Discreet notifications**: Receive personal information, such as messages or reminders, without having to consult a separate device.

4. **Increased autonomy**

    - **Independence in daily tasks**: Reduced dependence on others for activities such as managing finances, reading the mail or taking medication.
    - **Increased confidence**: Sense of security and autonomy thanks to direct access to information.

Examples of smart glasses for the blind

1. **OrCam MyEye**

    - **Description**: Compact device that attaches to the temples of eyeglasses. It uses a smart camera to read text, recognize faces, products and colors.
    - **Features** :

- Real-time reading of printed and digital texts.
- Recognition of pre-recorded faces.
- Product identification via barcodes.
- Offline operation, preserving data confidentiality.

2. **eSight**

    - **Description**: Electronic glasses for the visually impaired, combining high-definition cameras and OLED screens in front of the eyes.
    - **Features** :
        - Real-time image amplification.
        - Customized adjustments for sharpness, contrast and color.
        - Photos and videos can be taken.
        - Help with activities such as reading, working on the computer or watching TV.

3. **IrisVision**

    - **Description**: Device using a smartphone inserted into a modified virtual reality headset, designed for people with low vision.
    - **Features** :
        - Powerful optical zoom.
        - Customizable viewing modes for different eye conditions.
        - Access to applications and the Internet.

4. **Aira**

    - **Description**: Service combining smart glasses and remote human assistance.
    - **Features** :
        - Connection with live agents who describe the environment, read out information, and assist the user with various tasks.
        - Flexible use via glasses or smartphone.

Limitations and challenges of smart glasses

1. **High cost**
   - **Affordability**: The price of these devices can be prohibitive for many people. Financial aid is therefore essential to facilitate access.

2. **Learning and adaptation**
   - **Complexity of use**: training is often required to master the functions and get the most out of the device.
   - **Technological acceptance**: Some users may be reluctant to adopt new technologies.

3. **Comfort and aesthetics**
   - **Ergonomics**: The weight and size of devices can affect comfort during prolonged use.
   - **Discretion**: Some users prefer discreet solutions to avoid drawing attention to their disability.

4. **Dependence on connectivity**
   - **Internet connection**: Some functions, such as data updates and remote assistance, require a stable connection.

5. **Privacy and security**
   - **Data protection** : The information captured can be sensitive. It is important that devices guarantee the confidentiality and security of personal data.

The role of the caregiver in supporting the use of smart glasses

1. **Information and awareness-raising**
   - **Presentation of options**: Inform the patient about the different technologies available, explaining the advantages and limitations of each.
   - **Needs assessment**: To help determine which device best matches the patient's needs, abilities and goals.

2. **Assistance with administrative formalities**
   - **Finding financial aid**: help identify possible sources of funding, such as the Prestation de Compensation du Handicap (PCH), subsidies from associations or specific programs.
   - **File preparation**: Help patients prepare the documents they need to apply for assistance.

3. **Training and technical support**
   - **Training organization**: Put patients in touch with professionals or specialized centers for appropriate training.
   - **Installation assistance**: Helping to configure the device, customize settings and resolve technical problems.
   - **Encouraging practice**: Encourage patients to use their eyewear regularly, so that they feel more at ease.

4. **Emotional support**

    ○ **Managing apprehension**: Listen to the patient's fears or misgivings about the new technology, and offer empathetic support.
    ○ **Valuing progress**: Highlight successes and benefits to boost self-confidence.

5. **Coordination with healthcare professionals**

    ○ **Interdisciplinary collaboration**: Working closely with ophthalmologists, occupational therapists, locomotion instructors and technicians to ensure comprehensive care.
    ○ **Keeping** abreast **of** technological advances and updates to provide up-to-date support.

Future prospects and innovations

1. **Technology enhancement**

    ○ **Miniaturization**: Reducing the size and weight of devices for greater comfort.
    ○ **Advanced artificial intelligence**: more powerful algorithms for faster, more accurate recognition.
    ○ **Energy autonomy**: longer-lasting batteries and optimized energy management systems.

2. **Augmented reality integration**

    ○ **Immersive experiences**: the ability to add contextual information in real time, such as directions and descriptions of complex environments.
    ○ **Voice and gesture interaction**: control devices by voice or simple gestures for intuitive operation.

3. **Greater affordability**

    ○ **Lower production costs**: thanks to technological advances and the democratization of components.
    ○ **Expanded subsidy programs**: sensitize public and private institutions to provide financial support for the acquisition of these technologies.

4. **Customization and adaptation**

    ○ **Tailor-made solutions**: Development of devices adapted to the specific needs of each user, taking into account their degree of visual impairment, their habits and their environment.
    ○ **Compatibility with other technologies**: Integration with smartphones, navigation applications and home automation systems for a connected experience.

Vision rehabilitation technologies

- **Retinal implants and visual prostheses**

Vision loss is one of the most devastating afflictions that can affect an individual, profoundly impacting their quality of life, independence and participation in society. For decades, medicine and technology have been joining forces to find innovative solutions to restore, at least partially, vision in people suffering from blindness or severe visual impairment. Among these advances, retinal implants and visual prostheses represent a glimmer of hope, opening the way to new therapeutic possibilities. These high-tech devices, which combine biomedical engineering, neuroscience and microelectronics, aim to replace or stimulate failing structures in the eye or visual system, giving patients the ability to perceive visual stimuli again.

Understanding vision and its disturbances

To understand how retinal implants work, it's essential to understand the complex process of vision. The retina, located at the back of the eye, is a thin layer of nerve tissue that converts light into electrical signals. These signals are then transmitted to the brain via the optic nerve, where they are interpreted as images. Degenerative diseases of the retina, such as retinitis pigmentosa or age-related macular degeneration (AMD), damage the photoreceptors (light-sensitive cells), leading to progressive vision loss.

In many cases, even when photoreceptors are destroyed, other retinal neurons and visual pathways remain intact. This observation has led researchers to envisage solutions for directly stimulating these residual cells, thus bypassing the failing photoreceptors.

Retinal implants: an innovative approach

Retinal implants are electronic devices surgically implanted in the eye, designed to replace the functions of damaged photoreceptors. They fall into two main categories:

1. **Epiretinal implants**: Placed on the inner surface of the retina.
2. **Sub-retinal implants**: inserted under the retina, where the photoreceptors are located.

The Argus II system: a pioneer in epiretinal implants

The Argus II system, developed by US company Second Sight, is one of the best-known retinal implants, and was the first to receive regulatory approval for clinical use. Here's how it works:

- **External components**: A miniature camera integrated into a pair of glasses captures images of the environment. These images are processed by a portable processing unit, which converts the visual information into electronic signals.
- **Wireless transmission**: Processed signals are transmitted wirelessly to the retinal implant.
- **Retinal stimulation**: The implant, consisting of a matrix of electrodes placed on the retina, directly stimulates the remaining retinal ganglion cells, sending out electrical impulses corresponding to the images captured.
- **Visual perception**: Electrical signals are routed to the brain via the optic nerve, where they are interpreted as light perceptions.

Clinical results and patient benefits

Patients fitted with the Argus II implant have reported a significant improvement in their visual perception. Although the restored vision is not comparable to normal vision, it generally enables them to distinguish shapes, movements, and in some cases, to read large letters or recognize large objects. These improvements can have a profound impact on patients' independence and quality of life, enabling them to perform everyday tasks such as :

- **Obstacle detection**: avoid obstacles when walking, improving mobility and safety.
- **Shape recognition**: Identify the contours of objects, facilitating activities such as sorting clothes or preparing meals.
- **Social interaction**: Perceive people's movements, which helps in social interactions.

Sub-retinal implants: the example of the Alpha AMS device

The Alpha AMS device, developed by German company Retina Implant AG, is a subretinal implant designed to directly replace failing photoreceptors. It operates as follows:

- **Energy autonomy**: Unlike the Argus II, the Alpha AMS is powered by ambient light, thanks to integrated photodiodes that convert light into electrical signals.
- **Direct stimulation**: Placed under the retina, it stimulates bipolar neurons, the cells located just after the photoreceptors in the visual transmission chain.
- **Results**: Patients reported improvements in contrast perception, pattern recognition and reading large words.

Current challenges and limitations

Despite promising advances, retinal implants present several challenges and limitations:

- **Limited resolution**: The number of electrodes in current implants is relatively low, which limits the resolution of perceived images.
- **Cerebral adaptation**: the brain must learn to interpret new visual information, which requires a period of re-education and can vary from one individual to another.
- **Surgical complexity**: Implantation requires delicate surgery, with associated risks such as infection or retinal detachment.
- **High costs**: The cost of devices and surgical procedures is high, limiting accessibility for many patients.
- **Disease progression**: Implants are most effective in patients with functional inner retinal neurons and optic nerves. In progressive diseases, these structures may also be affected over time.

Other approaches to visual prostheses

In addition to retinal implants, other strategies are being explored to restore vision:

1. **Cortical implants**: These devices stimulate the brain's visual cortex directly. They are considered for patients with optic nerve damage.
2. **Optoelectronic implants**: using nanoparticles or light-sensitive polymers to make the remaining neurons sensitive to light.
3. **Gene therapy**: Introduction of genes coding for light-sensitive proteins (such as opsins) to restore light sensitivity to retinal cells.
4. **Stem cells**: Transplantation of stem cells to regenerate damaged photoreceptors.

Technological advances and future prospects

Research into retinal implants and visual prostheses is constantly evolving. Future prospects include :

- **Increased resolution**: Development of implants with a greater number of electrodes to improve the quality of the perceived image.
- **Advanced biocompatible materials**: Use of materials that reduce inflammatory reactions and increase implant longevity.
- **Improved wireless stimulation**: Technologies for transmitting signals and energy wirelessly, more efficiently and safely.
- **Artificial intelligence**: Integration of AI algorithms to optimize image processing and adapt stimulation to the specific needs of each patient.
- **Cost reduction**: Innovations in manufacturing processes to make devices more affordable.

The role of medical and paramedical support

Implanting a visual prosthesis is more than just a surgical procedure. Multidisciplinary support is essential to maximize the benefits for the patient:

- **Preoperative assessment**: Determine patient eligibility, explain realistic expectations and implications of surgery.
- **Visual rehabilitation**: Training program to teach patients to interpret new visual perceptions, often in collaboration with orthoptists and occupational therapists.
- **Psychological support**: Helping patients manage the emotions associated with partial vision recovery, and adapt to the changes in their daily lives.
- **Long-term follow-up**: Monitor eye health and implant function, and make any necessary adjustments.

Ethical and social considerations

The introduction of invasive technologies to restore vision also raises ethical questions:

- **Informed consent**: Patients must be fully informed of the risks, potential benefits and uncertainties associated with the procedure.
- **Equity of access**: Ensuring that advances don't just benefit those who can afford them, but are accessible to all those who could benefit from them.
- **Realistic expectations**: Avoid creating false hopes, by clearly communicating the current limitations of technologies.

- **Gene therapies and biomedical advances**

Modern medicine is on the cusp of a major revolution thanks to gene therapies and biomedical advances. These innovations promise not only to treat hitherto incurable diseases, but also to transform our fundamental understanding of human biology. Gene therapies, in particular, offer the hope of correcting genetic defects at source, paving the way for more effective, personalized treatments. In a world where genetic and degenerative diseases affect millions of people, these advances represent a decisive turning point towards more precise, more humane medicine.

Understanding gene therapy

Gene therapy is a medical approach that aims to treat or prevent disease by modifying the expression of genes within a patient's cells. Rather than treating the symptoms of a disease, gene therapy directly addresses its genetic cause. It involves the introduction, deletion or modification of genetic material in cells to correct abnormalities or provide new cellular functions.

The main gene therapy strategies include:

1. **Functional gene addition**: Introduction of a healthy gene to compensate for the effect of a defective or missing gene.
2. **Inactivation of defective genes**: Use of techniques to "switch off" the expression of a defective gene that causes disease.
3. **Genome editing**: Direct modification of the genome's DNA sequence to correct a mutation.

Key technological advances

Several technological advances have propelled the field of gene therapy:

1. **Safe and effective viral vectors**: Modified viruses are often used to deliver genetic material to target cells. Vectors such as adeno-associated viruses (AAVs) and lentiviruses have been optimized to maximize the safety and efficiency of gene transmission.

2. **Genome editing technologies**: The emergence of the CRISPR-Cas9 tool has revolutionized the ability to modify the genome with unprecedented precision. This technology makes it possible to specifically target a DNA sequence and modify, delete or insert it.

3. **In vivo and ex vivo gene therapies**: In vivo approaches involve direct administration of the therapeutic vector into the body, while ex vivo approaches involve taking cells from the patient, genetically modifying them in the laboratory, and then reintroducing them.

Promising clinical applications

Several diseases have been successfully targeted by gene therapies, demonstrating the immense potential of this approach.

1. **Hematological disorders**

    - *Sickle cell anemia*: A genetic disease affecting the hemoglobin in red blood cells. Ex vivo gene therapies have made it possible to correct the genetic defect in hematopoietic stem cells, resulting in the production of healthy red blood cells.

- *Hemophilia*: Patients with hemophilia lack essential coagulation factors. In vivo gene therapies have been developed to introduce genes coding for these factors, significantly reducing bleeding episodes.

2. **Neurodegenerative diseases**

    - *Spinal muscular atrophy*: A disease that affects motor neurons, leading to progressive muscle weakness. Gene therapy has made it possible to introduce a functional copy of the missing SMN1 gene, significantly improving patients' survival and motor function.

3. **Hereditary blindness**

    - *Leber congenital amaurosis*: A form of childhood blindness caused by mutations in the RPE65 gene. A gene therapy has been approved to deliver a functional copy of this gene to retinal cells, partially restoring vision in some patients.

4. **Severe combined immunodeficiency (SCID)**

    - SCID patients suffer from severe immune system deficiency. Gene therapies have been used to correct genetic defects in immune stem cells, restoring normal immune function.

Challenges and considerations

Despite promising successes, several challenges remain in the field of gene therapy:

1. **Security**

    ◦ *Immune reactions*: The introduction of viral vectors or new genes can provoke undesirable immune responses, compromising treatment efficacy or causing side effects.

    ◦ *Insertional mutagenesis*: Random integration of genetic material can disrupt essential genes, increasing the risk of cancer or other abnormalities.

2. **Delivery efficiency**

    ◦ *Specific cell targeting*: It's crucial that the vector reaches the relevant target cells without affecting healthy cells.

    ◦ *Sustainable gene expression*: Ensuring that the introduced gene remains active over the long term to provide ongoing therapeutic benefit.

3. **High costs**

    ◦ Gene therapies are often very expensive due to the complexity of their development and manufacture, limiting access for many patients.

4. **Ethical issues**

    ◦ *Genetic manipulation*: Intervention on the human genome raises ethical concerns, particularly as regards modifications that can be passed on to future generations.

    ◦ *Equity of access*: Ensuring that advances do not create additional disparities between different populations.

Related biomedical advances

In addition to gene therapy, other biomedical advances are helping to transform the medical landscape:

1. **Cellular therapies**

    - *Induced pluripotent stem (iPS) cells*: These cells, reprogrammed from adult cells, can differentiate into any cell type, opening up possibilities for tissue regeneration and disease modeling.

    - *Cellular immunotherapies*: the patient's own immune cells can be modified to specifically target cancer cells, as in CAR-T therapies for certain types of leukemia.

2. **Nanomedicine**

    - *Nanoparticles for drug delivery*: These particles can carry drugs directly to diseased cells, improving efficacy and reducing side effects.

    - *Nanodiagnostics*: Use of nanotechnologies for early detection of diseases at the molecular level.

3. **Advanced genome editing**

    - *Improved CRISPR techniques*: Development of more precise and safer variants, such as CRISPR-Cas13 for RNA editing, reducing the risk of off-target modifications.

4. **Personalized medicine**

    - *Genetic profiling*: Using individual genetic information to tailor treatments, optimizing their effectiveness and minimizing side effects.

- *Biomarkers*: Identification of biological markers for early diagnosis, disease monitoring and prediction of response to treatment.

The future of gene therapy and biomedical advances

The potential of gene therapy and biomedical advances is immense, and the future promises even more revolutionary developments:

1. **Treatment of common illnesses**

    - Expanding applications to include non-genetic diseases, such as cardiovascular disease or diabetes, by modulating the expression of the genes involved.

2. **Genomic editing in utero**

    - Intervening before birth to correct serious genetic anomalies, offering early disease prevention.

3. **Combination therapies**

    - Integrating gene therapy with other approaches, such as immunotherapy, for more comprehensive and effective treatments.

4. **Vector enhancement**

    - Development of non-viral vectors, such as lipid nanoparticles, for safer, more targeted delivery.

5. **Ethics and regulations**

    - Establishment of robust ethical and regulatory frameworks to oversee advances, ensuring responsible research and safe clinical application.

The role of healthcare professionals

Healthcare professionals, including caregivers, have a crucial role to play in this new medical era:

1. **Education and information**
   - Inform patients and their families about treatment options, potential benefits and associated risks.

2. **Emotional support**
   - Accompany patients on their journey, understanding the hopes and concerns associated with these innovative therapies.

3. **Care coordination**
   - Work with a multidisciplinary team to ensure comprehensive care, including medical, psychological and social aspects.

4. **Scientific watch**
   - Keeping abreast of the latest advances to offer care at the cutting edge of technology and participating in the dissemination of knowledge.

- **Virtual reality in rehabilitation**

Virtual reality (VR) is an immersive technology that simulates an artificial environment, often in three dimensions, in which users can interact realistically. It has transformed many fields, and rehabilitation is a particularly significant example. By offering personalized, interactive experiences, VR is revolutionizing traditional approaches to rehabilitation, whether physical, cognitive or psychological.

The benefits of virtual reality in rehabilitation

The integration of virtual reality into rehabilitation programs offers multiple benefits, improving the effectiveness of treatments and the well-being of patients.

1. **Enhanced patient engagement**
   The immersive nature of VR captures patients' attention, immersing them in stimulating environments that make rehabilitation exercises more engaging. This engagement encourages active and regular participation, essential for significant progress.

2. **Personalized therapies**
   VR makes it possible to create scenarios tailored to the specific needs of each patient. Therapists can adjust task difficulty, exercise types and virtual environments to suit individual goals, optimizing results.

3. **Safe practice environment**
   Patients can practice in situations that would be difficult or risky in the real world. For example, a person relearning to walk can navigate in a virtual space without fear of falling, boosting confidence and speeding recovery.

4. **Motivation and treatment adherence**
   The fun, interactive aspects of VR transform rehabilitation sessions into enjoyable experiences. Patients are more inclined to follow their therapy program, which improves adherence and overall treatment efficacy.

Virtual reality applications in various fields of rehabilitation

VR is used in a variety of therapeutic contexts, offering innovative solutions for different types of rehabilitation.

1. **Motor rehabilitation**
   For patients who have suffered a stroke, brain injury or neurological disorder, VR helps to relearn movement and restore motor function.
   - **Coordination and balance exercises**: Patients can take part in virtual activities that stimulate hand-eye coordination, balance and posture.
   - **Real-time feedback**: VR systems provide immediate feedback on performance, enabling patients to correct their movements and therapists to monitor progress.

2. **Cognitive rehabilitation**
   VR is used to improve cognitive functions such as memory, attention, planning and problem-solving.
   - **Cognitive stimulation games**: Virtual environments offer tasks that challenge working memory, concentration and mental flexibility.
   - **Simulation of real-life situations**: Patients can practice everyday activities, such as shopping or managing finances, in a controlled setting.

3. **Psychological rehabilitation**
   VR offers innovative approaches to treating psychological disorders, including phobias, post-traumatic stress disorder (PTSD) and anxiety.
   - **Exposure therapy**: Patients are gradually exposed to anxiety-provoking stimuli in a safe environment, helping to reduce fear reactions.

- **Stress management**: Soothing environments are used to teach relaxation and emotional management techniques.

4. **Pain management**

   VR can distract patients from acute or chronic pain, by reducing the perception of pain.

   - **Immersion in soothing environments**: Patients are immersed in relaxing virtual landscapes, reducing the intensity of the pain they feel.
   - **Interactive games**: Focusing on engaging tasks diverts attention away from pain.

Examples of VR rehabilitation technologies and programs

1. **Adapted VR devices**

   - **Virtual reality headsets**: Devices like the Oculus Rift, HTC Vive or PlayStation VR are used to create immersive experiences.
   - **Motion sensors**: Devices such as the Kinect or haptic gloves can track the patient's movements and interact with the virtual environment.

2. **Specific programs**

   - **Virtual Rehab**: A platform offering motor and cognitive rehabilitation exercises, with customizable programs.
   - **MindMaze**: Using VR and mixed reality to aid neurological recovery after stroke or brain injury.
   - **SnowWorld**: A virtual environment designed for pain management in burn patients.

Challenges and limitations of using VR in rehabilitation

Despite its many advantages, integrating VR into rehabilitation presents certain challenges.

1. **Accessibility and cost**

    - **High initial investment**: The cost of equipment and software can be prohibitive for certain care facilities or for home use.
    - **Staff training**: Therapists need to be trained in the use of these technologies, which requires time and resources.

2. **Tailored to individual needs**

    - **Limited personalization**: Not all programs allow for fine-tuning to the specific needs of each patient.
    - **Comfort and tolerance**: Some patients may experience discomfort, such as simulator sickness or headaches.

3. **Technical constraints**

    - **Equipment reliability**: Devices can experience technical problems, interrupting rehabilitation sessions.
    - **Upgrades and maintenance**: Systems need to be kept up to date to ensure proper operation.

The role of healthcare professionals in integrating VR

Healthcare professionals play an essential role in the adoption and effectiveness of VR in rehabilitation.

1. **Training and skills**
    - **Technology mastery**: Therapists need to be familiar with equipment and software in order to use them effectively.
    - **Interdisciplinary approach**: collaboration between doctors, physiotherapists, occupational therapists and engineers to optimize rehabilitation programs.

2. **Monitoring and adjusting therapies**
    - **Progress assessment**: Using data provided by VR systems to monitor progress and adjust therapeutic goals.
    - **Program adaptation**: Modify exercises according to the patient's response to maximize benefits.

3. **Patient support**
    - **Managing expectations**: Inform the patient about realistic goals and possible limitations of VR.
    - **Psychological support**: to help the patient overcome any frustrations or obstacles encountered when using the technology.

Future prospects for virtual reality in rehabilitation

Technological advances continue to expand the possibilities offered by VR in rehabilitation.

1. **Integrating artificial intelligence**
    - **Greater personalization**: AI can analyze patient data to automatically adapt exercises and virtual environments.

- **Outcome prediction**: Use of predictive models to anticipate progress and adjust therapies accordingly.

2. **Augmented and mixed reality**

    - **Enriching the real environment**: Augmented reality superimposes virtual information on the real world, enabling more natural rehabilitation exercises.
    - **Social interaction**: work in groups or with avatars, enhancing motivation and commitment.

3. **Improved accessibility**

    - **Wearable technologies**: Development of lighter, less expensive devices, making them easier to use at home.
    - **Mobile applications**: Rehabilitation programs accessible via smartphones or tablets, extending the reach of therapies.

Integrating technology into daily care

- **Training nurses in the use of new technologies**

Rapidly evolving technologies have profoundly transformed the landscape of the healthcare sector, opening up new opportunities to improve patient care and support. Caregivers, on the front line in the day-to-day care of vulnerable people, must adapt to these changes to maintain a high level of quality in their interventions. Training in the use of new technologies is therefore no longer an option, but an imperative necessity to meet the current and future challenges facing the profession.

Caregivers play a crucial role in supporting patients, particularly those with visual impairments. Assistive technologies, such as screen-reading applications, electronic walking sticks, adapted GPS navigation systems or object and text recognition software, are now indispensable tools for promoting the autonomy and social inclusion of blind or partially-sighted people. However, for these technologies to be fully effective, it is essential that the professionals who work with these patients are trained in their use.

The training of healthcare assistants must begin with an awareness of the challenges posed by new technologies in the healthcare field. The aim is to understand how these tools can improve patients' quality of life, reduce their dependency and facilitate their integration into society. This awareness is the first step towards effective appropriation of technologies.

Secondly, training must be practical and focused on the practical use of technological devices. Caregivers need to be able to configure devices, install applications, customize settings according to the specific needs of each patient, and solve common technical problems. For example, knowing how to guide a patient through the use of a screen-reading application requires a thorough understanding of the software's functionalities, voice or gesture commands, and methods for optimizing accessibility.

It is also important that training courses incorporate real-life situations, enabling caregivers to practice with patients in a safe environment. This hands-on approach fosters the acquisition of operational skills and reinforces the confidence of professionals in their ability to accompany patients effectively. For example, accompanying a patient on an outing using an adapted GPS navigation system enables the caregiver to master the particularities of the device, while assessing the patient's reactions in a real-life situation.

At the same time, training must include a component on the ethical and regulatory aspects of using healthcare technologies. Caregivers need to be aware of the issues of confidentiality, personal data protection and the legal limits associated with certain devices. Understanding these aspects is essential to ensure responsible use that respects patients' rights.

Ongoing training is another key element. Technologies evolve rapidly, with new applications, updates and innovations appearing regularly. Caregivers must therefore have access to regular training programs to keep abreast of the latest advances. Healthcare establishments and training organizations have a major role to play in offering refresher sessions, practical workshops and online resources.

It is also beneficial to encourage the exchange of best practices between professionals. Caregivers can learn a lot from their peers, by sharing experiences, challenges and solutions. Communities of practice, online forums and professional networks are ideal platforms for such exchanges.

Finally, it is essential to recognize and promote the technological skills acquired by caregivers. This can be achieved by certifying training courses, integrating these skills into professional assessments, and promoting these skills to patients and their families. Such recognition helps to motivate professionals and underscore the importance of their role in providing technological support for patients.

- **Helping patients adopt technology**

The integration of technology into healthcare has revolutionized the way care is delivered, offering new opportunities to improve patients' quality of life. However, the adoption of these technologies by patients can be a complex process, requiring tailored support to ensure effective and beneficial use. Accompanying patients in this process is therefore essential to overcome potential obstacles and maximize the benefits of technological innovations.

The adoption of technology by patients has many benefits, such as empowerment, improved communication with healthcare professionals, and better monitoring of their health status. Nevertheless, several factors can hinder this adoption, including unfamiliarity with technologies, fear of the unknown, lack of digital skills, or concerns about data confidentiality.

The role of healthcare professionals in providing support

Healthcare professionals, particularly nursing assistants, play a crucial role in helping patients to adopt technology. Their proximity to patients and in-depth knowledge of their needs and concerns make them key players in this process.

1. **Assessing needs and capabilities**
   It's important to start with a personalized assessment of the patient's needs, technological capabilities and any apprehensions. This step helps to determine which technologies are most suitable, and how they can be gradually integrated into the patient's daily life.

2. **Information and awareness**
   Patients need to be informed of the benefits that technologies can bring them, in terms of autonomy, comfort and quality of life. It is essential to present the tools in a positive light, emphasizing their practical usefulness and dispelling any fears associated with their use.

3. **Customized training**
   Training adapted to the patient's skill level is essential to ensure effective appropriation of the technologies. This training must be practical, interactive and focused on the functionalities most relevant to the patient. It can include demonstrations, guided exercises and the provision of accessible teaching aids.

4. **Ongoing support and follow-up**
   Support doesn't stop with initial training. Ongoing

support is crucial to help patients overcome any difficulties they may encounter. This means being available to answer questions, offering refresher sessions if necessary, and monitoring the use of technologies to ensure they are meeting the patient's expectations.

5. **Adaptation and personalization**
   Technologies need to be adapted to the specific needs and preferences of each patient. This may involve customizing parameters, selecting the most appropriate applications or devices, and adjusting the user environment to maximize comfort and efficiency.

Strategies to facilitate technology adoption

1. **Involving the patient in the decision-making process**
   It's important for patients to feel that they have a stake in their own technological journey. Involving them in the choice of tools and methods strengthens their commitment and motivation to use them.

2. **Use clear, accessible language**
   When explaining, it's essential to avoid technical jargon and use simple, understandable language. Analogies with familiar situations can help clarify complex concepts.

3. **Creating a reassuring learning environment**
   Learning needs to take place in a caring environment, where the patient feels comfortable asking questions and expressing difficulties. Patience and encouragement are key to building this confidence.

4. **Highlighting concrete examples**
   Illustrating the benefits of technology through concrete examples that are relevant to the patient can facilitate understanding and arouse interest. For example, show

how a medication reminder application can help patients better manage their treatment.

5. **Encouraging experimentation**
Encouraging patients to explore technologies on their own, while being available to guide them, fosters autonomy and confidence in their own abilities.

Managing obstacles and resistance

Patients often express resistance to new technologies. This resistance may be linked to fears, negative past experiences, or a feeling of not being able to learn. To deal with these obstacles :

1. **Listening to and understanding concerns**
Taking the time to listen to the patient's concerns allows us to address them in a specific way. It's important to acknowledge these feelings without judgment.

2. **Offering customized solutions**
Offer alternatives or adjustments to address patient concerns, such as devices with simplified interfaces or enhanced safety options.

3. **Celebrating small victories**
Celebrating progress, however modest, boosts patients' confidence and encourages them to continue their efforts.

4. **Involving family and friends**
Family and friends can play an important support role. Including them in the process can help create a favorable environment for technology adoption.

The importance of data confidentiality and security

Concerns about confidentiality and data security are legitimate and must be taken into account. It is essential to inform patients of the safeguards in place, to explain how their data is used, and to give them advice on how to keep their personal information secure.

The role of continuing education for professionals

To support patients effectively, caregivers themselves need to be trained in the technologies they present. Ongoing training enables them to keep abreast of the latest innovations, develop their technical skills and learn appropriate teaching methods.

- **Data security and confidentiality**

In an increasingly connected world, data security and confidentiality have become major concerns for individuals, businesses and governments alike. The rise of information and communication technologies has transformed the way we live, work and communicate, but it has also created new risks linked to the protection of personal and sensitive information. Data security is no longer limited to protection against computer viruses or unauthorized intrusion; it now encompasses a complex set of technical, legal and ethical challenges that require a global, proactive approach.

The challenges of data security

Data security aims to protect information from unauthorized access, disclosure, modification or destruction. Threats can come from a variety of sources, such as cyber-attacks, malware, human error or technical failures. The consequences of a security breach can be devastating:

1. **Loss of critical data**: The destruction or corruption of essential data can paralyze an organization's activities, resulting in considerable financial losses.

2. **Reputation damage**: Security incidents can damage the trust of customers, partners and the public, with lasting effects on brand image.

3. **Legal liability**: Companies can be held responsible for security breaches, with financial and legal penalties.

4. **Industrial espionage**: Sensitive information can be stolen for purposes of unfair competition or economic sabotage.

The fundamentals of data security

To meet these challenges, it is essential to adopt an approach based on the fundamental principles of information security:

1. **Confidentiality**: Ensuring that information is only accessible to authorized persons. This involves the use of access controls, encryption and identity management policies.

2. **Integrity**: Ensuring that data is accurate and has not been altered in an unauthorized way. Integrity control mechanisms, such as digital signatures and hashes, are used for this purpose.

3. **Availability**: Ensuring that information and systems are accessible to authorized users when they need them. This requires measures to prevent outages, denial-of-service attacks and other disruptions.

4. **Traceability**: Record activities and accesses to enable auditing and the detection of abnormal or malicious behavior.

The challenges of data confidentiality

Data privacy concerns the right of individuals to control the use and disclosure of their personal information. Key challenges include:

1. **Massive data collection**: Companies collect large amounts of data for commercial reasons, such as targeted marketing or service improvement. This raises questions about the purpose of the collection and the consent of individuals.

2. **Data sharing and transfer**: Personal data is often shared between different entities, sometimes without individuals' knowledge or explicit consent.

3. **Storage and retention**: How data is stored and for how long raises issues of security and regulatory compliance.

4. **Profiling and discrimination**: Using data to profile individuals can lead to discriminatory or intrusive practices.

Legislative and regulatory frameworks

To protect personal data, many countries have implemented strict laws and regulations. One of the most significant examples is the European Union's General Data Protection Regulation (GDPR), which came into force in May 2018. The RGPD sets high standards for the protection of personal data and imposes obligations on organizations that process such data, including:

1. **Explicit consent**: Organizations must obtain clear and informed consent from individuals before collecting or using their data.

2. **Right of access and rectification**: Individuals have the right to access their personal data and request corrections in the event of inaccuracy.

3. **Right to be forgotten** : Individuals may request the deletion of their data under certain conditions.

4. **Breach notification**: In the event of a data breach, organizations must inform the competent authorities and the individuals concerned as soon as possible.

5. **Transparency**: Companies must be transparent about how they collect, process and store data.

Best practices for security and confidentiality

To comply with regulations and effectively protect data, organizations must adopt appropriate technical and organizational measures:

1. **Establish security policies**: Draw up clear policies defining responsibilities, procedures and security protocols.

2. **Staff training**: Make employees aware of data security risks and best practices.

3. **Use of encryption** : Protect data in transit and at rest using robust encryption techniques.

4. **Strict access controls**: Limit access to data to only those who need it for their work, using strong authentication and well-defined authorizations.

5. **Vulnerability management**: Perform regular scans to identify and correct system weaknesses.

6. **Incident response plan** : Prepare a plan to respond quickly and effectively in the event of a security breach.

7. **Privacy Impact Assessment**: Performing analyses to understand how data processing affects the privacy of individuals and to minimize risks.

Emerging technologies and their implications

Technological advances such as artificial intelligence, the Internet of Things (IoT) and cloud computing present new opportunities, but also new challenges for data security and confidentiality:

1. **Artificial Intelligence (AI)**: AI can process large amounts of data to provide advanced analytics, but it requires access to potentially sensitive data. It is crucial to ensure that algorithms are transparent and that data is used ethically.

2. **Internet of Things (IoT)**: Connected devices are constantly collecting and exchanging data, increasing the potential attack surface. Security must be integrated into the design of these devices.

3. **Cloud computing**: Storing and processing data on remote servers requires trust in cloud service providers and measures to guarantee data security in a shared environment.

Shared responsibility

Data security and confidentiality are not just the responsibility of organizations; individuals also have a role to play:

1. **Risk awareness**: Users should be aware of the risks involved in disclosing their personal information, and adopt a cautious attitude.

2. **Password management**: Using strong, unique passwords, and changing them regularly, is essential to protect access to your data.

3. **Software updates**: Keep devices and applications up-to-date to benefit from security patches.

4. **Privacy settings**: check and adjust privacy settings on social networks and applications to control what information is shared.

Chapter 9

Integrating family and caregivers

The family's role in the care process

- **Emotional and practical support**

Emotional and practical support is a fundamental element in the care of blind and partially-sighted people. Loss of vision, whether progressive or sudden, brings with it considerable challenges that affect not only the ability to perform daily tasks, but also psychological well-being and social integration. Understanding the importance of this support, and knowing how to provide it effectively, is essential to helping these people overcome obstacles, develop their independence and live fulfilling lives.

The emotional impact of vision loss

Blindness or low vision can trigger a range of intense emotions, such as shock, denial, anger, sadness and anxiety. These feelings are often associated with mourning the loss of an essential sense and uncertainty about the future. Those affected may experience :

- **Decreased self-esteem**: The perception of no longer being able to perform once-simple tasks can affect self-confidence.
- **Social isolation**: Difficulty getting around or taking part in social activities can lead to withdrawal and increased loneliness.
- **Increased dependence**: The need for help with daily activities can lead to a feeling of loss of control and independence.

It is therefore crucial to recognize these emotions and provide appropriate support to help people deal with them constructively.

The role of emotional support

Emotional support aims to help individuals cope with the psychological challenges associated with vision loss. It includes:

1. **Active listening**
   Offering an attentive ear enables people to express their feelings and concerns freely. It involves :
   - **Show empathy**: Understand and share other people's emotions without judgment.
   - **Validating feelings**: Recognize the legitimacy of the emotions you feel, whether sadness, frustration or fear.
   - **Encourage expression**: Invite people to talk about their experiences and needs.

2. **Professional psychological support**
   Psychologists, counsellors and specialized therapists can help :
   - **Develop coping strategies**: Learn techniques to manage stress, anxiety and emotional changes.
   - **Reinforce self-esteem**: Work on self-perception and confidence in one's abilities.
   - **Preventing depression**: Identifying early signs and intervening to avoid a deterioration in mental health.

3. **Family and social support**
   Family and friends play an essential role in :
   - **Providing a secure environment**: Providing a reassuring presence and constant support.
   - **Encouraging autonomy**: Helping without over-protecting, allowing the person to make their own experiences.

- **Facilitating communication**: Maintaining social interaction to prevent isolation.

The role of practical support

Practical support aims to help blind and partially-sighted people acquire the skills and resources they need to live independently. It includes :

1. **Life skills training**

    - **Braille learning**: Enabling reading and writing for access to information and education.
    - **Mobility techniques**: Teaching the use of the white cane, spatial orientation and safe movement techniques.
    - **Home management**: Learn how to cook, manage household chores and use household appliances appropriately.

2. **Access to assistive technologies**

    - **Electronic devices**: Use screen readers, adapted mobile applications and hearing aids.
    - **Specialized equipment**: Install devices such as beacons, Braille keyboards or talking watches.
    - **User training**: Support in mastering these tools and integrating them into daily life.

3. **Adapting the environment**

    - **Home design**: Modify furniture layout, install appropriate lighting for the visually impaired, use tactile cues.
    - **Accessibility in public spaces**: Promote adapted infrastructures, such as audible crosswalks and elevators with Braille signage.

- **Adapted signage**: Use color contrasts, enlarged characters and pictograms to facilitate orientation.

4. **Support with administrative formalities**
    - **Access to rights and benefits**: Help with applications for benefits, financial aid and support services.
    - **Referral to specialized services**: Put you in touch with associations, rehabilitation centers and relevant professionals.
    - **Legal support**: Information on employment, housing and non-discrimination rights.

The role of healthcare professionals and caregivers

Healthcare professionals, including doctors, nurses, carers and social workers, have a key responsibility in providing emotional and practical support:

- **Comprehensive needs assessment**: Identify medical, psychological and social needs to draw up a personalized support plan.
- **Service coordination**: Working with a multidisciplinary team to ensure coherent, effective care.
- **Training and information**: Provide clear information on treatment options, available resources and coping strategies.
- **Empathy and respect**: Treat each person with dignity, respecting their choices and valuing their skills.

The importance of support groups and social networks

Support groups provide a space where blind or partially sighted people can share their experiences, exchange advice and feel understood:

- **A stronger sense of belonging**: Feeling that you're not alone in the face of challenges can boost morale and motivation.
- **Information sharing**: Learn from others about effective strategies, useful technologies and available resources.
- **Creating social ties**: Developing friendships and relationships that enrich everyday life.

Promoting autonomy and inclusion

Emotional and practical support ultimately aims to enable blind and partially-sighted people to lead as independent and fulfilling a life as possible. This involves:

- **Encourage active participation**: Encourage involvement in educational, professional, cultural and recreational activities.
- **Combating stereotypes**: Raising society's awareness of the abilities and contributions of blind people, to reduce prejudice and discrimination.
- **Adapting environments**: Working with institutions, businesses and communities to create accessible and inclusive environments.

- **Collaboration with orderlies**

Collaboration with caregivers is a fundamental pillar of care for people who are blind or visually impaired. These healthcare professionals play a crucial role in day-to-day care, offering not only physical care, but also emotional and social support. Their commitment goes beyond traditional tasks, as they actively contribute to patients' autonomy, social integration and general well-being. Understanding the importance of this collaboration, and putting in place effective strategies to strengthen it, is essential to improving the quality of life of those concerned.

The essential role of orderlies

Care assistants are key players in the healthcare system, working directly with patients to meet their immediate needs. In the context of visual impairment, their role covers several aspects:

1. **Assistance with daily activities**
   Caregivers help patients with the essential tasks of daily living, such as washing, dressing, preparing meals and taking medication. Their presence not only ensures patients' physical safety, but also boosts their self-confidence, encouraging them to take an active part in these activities.

2. **Emotional and psychological support**
   Vision loss can lead to feelings of frustration, sadness and isolation. Caregivers listen attentively, offer encouragement and help patients express and manage their emotions. Their empathy and understanding are valuable assets in helping patients overcome the psychological challenges associated with their condition.

3. **Promoting independence**
   The main objective is to promote patients' independence. Caregivers encourage them to develop new skills, use technical aids and adopt coping strategies. They take care not to do things for the patient, but to guide them so that they can do them themselves.

4. **Education and training**
   They play an educational role by informing patients about available resources, assistive technologies and techniques to facilitate their daily lives. They can also train patients in the use of specific devices, such as screen readers or electronic canes.

The benefits of closer collaboration

Close collaboration between patients, caregivers and other healthcare professionals has many advantages:

1. **Patient-centred approach**
   By working together, we can develop a personalized care plan that takes into account the patient's specific needs, preferences and goals. This holistic approach promotes more effective and respectful care for the individual.

2. **Improved communication**
   Fluid communication between all parties enables relevant information to be shared, problems to be anticipated and interventions to be coordinated. Caregivers often act as a link between patients, their families and the medical team, facilitating exchanges and mutual understanding.

3. **Early detection of problems**
   Thanks to their regular presence with patients, caregivers are able to spot changes in health or behavior at an early stage. This vigilance enables them to intervene quickly when necessary, avoiding complications or unnecessary hospitalization.

4. **Support for social integration**
   Collaboration with caregivers encourages patients to take part in social, cultural and professional activities. They can accompany patients on outings, help them familiarize themselves with new environments and encourage them to maintain social ties.

The key components of effective collaboration

For collaboration to be successful, several elements must be present:

1. **Mutual trust**
   The relationship between patient and caregiver must be based on trust. This implies respect for confidentiality, reliability in actions and a caring attitude. Trust enables the patient to feel secure and to freely express his or her needs and concerns.

2. **Open communication**
   Open and honest communication is essential. Caregivers need to listen to patients, use clear and appropriate language, and regularly check mutual understanding. They must also be attentive to non-verbal cues and adapt their approach accordingly.

3. **Training and skills**
   Caregivers must have the necessary skills to effectively support blind or partially-sighted patients. This includes specific training in guiding techniques, adapted communication, the use of assistive technologies and the management of emergency situations.

4. **Interprofessional collaboration**
   Teamwork with other healthcare professionals is crucial. Care assistants must take part in coordination meetings, share their observations and contribute to the development of care plans. This synergy ensures coherent, comprehensive care.

The challenges ahead

Despite the many advantages, there are still obstacles to collaboration:

1. **Lack of resources**
   Budgetary constraints or staff shortages can limit the amount of time caregivers can devote to each patient. This can affect the quality of the relationship and the effectiveness of interventions.

2. **Communication barriers**
Communication difficulties may arise due to cultural or linguistic differences, or associated disorders (e.g. hearing loss). It's important to develop strategies to overcome these barriers.

3. **Resistance to change**
Some patients may be reluctant to accept help or adopt new methods. It is essential to respect their point of view, while gradually encouraging them to consider beneficial alternatives.

Strategies for strengthening collaboration

1. **Investment in training**
Offer caregivers ongoing training on the specificities of visual impairment, technological innovations and patient-centered approaches.

2. **Use of communication technologies**
Mobile applications, online platforms and secure messaging tools can facilitate communication between caregivers, patients and other members of the care team.

3. **Involving family and friends**
Working with the patient's family and friends can create a strong support network. Caregivers can train relatives in basic techniques and involve them in day-to-day activities.

4. **Adapting schedules and services**
Flexible schedules to better meet patients' individual needs, taking into account their lifestyle rhythms and preferences.

The importance of empathy and respect

At the heart of collaboration lies empathy. Caregivers must be able to put themselves in the patient's shoes, to understand their emotions and perspectives. Respect for the patient's autonomy and dignity is paramount. This means recognizing their rights, their choices and their desire to control their own lives.

Future prospects

With technological advances and changes in approaches to care, the role of care assistants is set to evolve. They will be increasingly involved in :

- **Support for the use of new technologies**: Helping patients master the digital tools that can enhance their autonomy.
- **Participation in rehabilitation programs**: Working with rehabilitation professionals to help patients develop new skills.
- **Health promotion**: raising patients' awareness of preventive measures and healthy lifestyle habits.

Communication and education of relatives

- **Provide clear information on the patient's condition**

Communication between healthcare professionals and patients is at the heart of effective, humanistic medical care. Providing clear information about the patient's condition is essential to establishing a relationship of trust, encouraging adherence to treatment and respecting the fundamental rights of individuals. This requires an empathetic approach, attentive listening and the adaptation of medical language to make it accessible to all.

The importance of clear communication in healthcare

Clarity in medical communication is essential for several reasons. Firstly, it enables patients to understand their condition, the issues involved and the treatment options available. This understanding is essential if they are to actively participate in decisions concerning their health, in line with the principle of informed consent. What's more, clear information reduces anxiety and uncertainty, giving patients a clearer picture of their situation.

Benefits for patients and healthcare professionals

Effective communication strengthens the therapeutic relationship. Patients feel respected and valued, which increases their confidence in the healthcare professional. This trust facilitates the exchange of information, enabling the caregiver to gather essential data for an accurate diagnosis. What's more, a well-informed patient is more likely to follow medical recommendations, improving clinical outcomes and reducing the risk of complications.

Adapting medical language to make it accessible

Medical jargon can be a major barrier to understanding for many patients. It is therefore crucial to translate technical terms into simple, clear language, while avoiding oversimplifications that could distort the information. It's useful to use analogies or concrete examples to illustrate complex concepts. For example, explaining how the heart works by comparing it to a pump can help to grasp its role in blood circulation.

Active listening and empathy

Active listening is an essential component of communication. It involves paying full attention to the patient, showing empathy and acknowledging emotions and concerns. By asking open-ended questions, the healthcare professional encourages the patient to express him/herself freely, enabling a better understanding of his/her needs and expectations. Empathy strengthens the therapeutic bond and shows patients that they are supported in their care.

Check the patient's understanding

After providing information, it's important to make sure the patient has understood. This can be done by asking them to rephrase in their own words what has been explained. This technique, known as "rephrasing", helps to identify points that may require further clarification. It avoids misunderstandings and ensures that the patient has all the information needed to make informed decisions.

Managing emotions and reactions

The announcement of a diagnosis or treatment can arouse strong emotions, such as fear, sadness or anger. The healthcare professional must be prepared to welcome these reactions with compassion. It's important to give patients time to express their feelings, and to answer their questions patiently. Offering emotional support can help patients come to terms with their condition and look forward to the next steps with greater serenity.

Involving the patient in decision-making

Active patient participation in decisions concerning their health is a key aspect of respecting their autonomy. By presenting the different treatment options, with their benefits and risks, the healthcare professional enables the patient to make informed choices. This collaboration strengthens the patient's commitment to his or her own care and can improve compliance with treatment.

Use visual and written aids

Visual aids, such as diagrams, images or videos, can help illustrate complex information. Similarly, providing clear, concise written documents enables patients to reread information at their own pace, and to share these documents with their loved ones. These materials should be written in accessible language and, if possible, adapted to the patient's literacy level.

Taking account of language and cultural barriers

In a multicultural society, it is common to encounter patients whose mother tongue is not that of the healthcare professional. Professional interpreters are essential to ensure effective communication. Moreover, being sensitive to cultural differences can help to adapt speech and avoid misunderstandings linked to the patient's values or beliefs.

Respecting the right to information and medical confidentiality

The right to information is a fundamental principle enshrined in legislation and professional ethics. Patients have the right to know about their state of health, proposed treatments and possible alternatives. At the same time, medical secrecy must be strictly respected, with information disclosed only with the patient's consent or in situations provided for by law.

Demonstrate availability

It is important that patients feel free to ask questions at any time. The healthcare professional must be available, whether during consultations or through other means of communication, to answer any questions that may arise afterwards. This availability reinforces trust and the feeling of being supported.

- **Training relatives in assistance techniques**

Loss of vision, whether gradual or sudden, represents a major upheaval in a person's life. Faced with this challenge, the support of loved ones is essential to promote the autonomy, well-being and social integration of the blind or partially-sighted person. However, to be truly effective, this support must be based on in-depth knowledge of assistive technologies specific to visual impairment. Training relatives in these techniques is therefore a crucial step that benefits both the person concerned and those around him or her. This training not only improves quality of life, but also strengthens family ties and friendships by fostering better mutual understanding.

The importance of training loved ones

Relatives play a central role in the day-to-day care of blind and partially-sighted people. Their involvement can facilitate adaptation to the new situation, encourage autonomy and prevent social isolation. However, without proper training, they may feel helpless, make mistakes or inadvertently hinder the development of the person's independence. The training aims to :

- **Providing practical tools**: Learning assistance techniques enables loved ones to help effectively without overprotecting or infantilizing the person.
- **Understanding specific needs**: A better understanding of the challenges faced by the visually impaired promotes empathy and communication.
- **Encouraging autonomy**: By mastering best practices, caregivers can support the learning of new skills and avoid creating excessive dependency.
- **Reduce stress and anxiety**: Training brings a certain serenity by giving clear guidelines on how to act in different situations.

Key training areas

1. **Guiding techniques**
   Learning how to guide a blind or partially-sighted person is fundamental to ensuring their safety when traveling. The course covers :

- **The correct position**: Stand slightly forward, offering your arm so that the person can hold it at elbow level.
- **Verbal directions**: Use clear descriptions to warn of changes in terrain, obstacles or steps.
- **Walking pace**: adapt your speed to that of the person you are guiding, making sure they feel at ease.
- **Narrow passages**: Point out narrow spaces by placing your arm behind your back so that the person comes up behind you.

2. **Appropriate communication**

The way we communicate has a significant impact on the quality of interactions:

- **Use precise language**: Avoid vague expressions such as "over there" or "here", preferring directional indications such as "to your right" or "three steps ahead".
- **Name those present**: In group conversations, mention who's present to facilitate participation.
- **Warn before you go**: Always inform the person you're going away, so they don't talk to someone who's no longer there.

3. **Environmental design**

Adapt living space to make it accessible and safe:

- **Maintain order**: keep objects in fixed places so that the person can find them easily.
- **Eliminate obstacles**: Avoid leaving objects lying around on the ground or in the path of travel.
- **Use tactile cues**: Install podotactile strips or different textures to signal room changes or areas at risk.

- **Optimize lighting**: For the visually impaired, adjusting light intensity and reducing glare can improve visual comfort.

4. **Use of assistive technologies**
   Relatives can be trained in the use of technological devices to better support the person:
   - **Mobile applications**: Learn how to set up and use screen-reading, object recognition and GPS navigation applications.
   - **Electronic devices**: Understand how Braille displays, audio players and electronic magnifiers work.
   - **Maintenance**: know how to maintain and troubleshoot equipment to keep it running smoothly.

5. **Emotional support**
   Beyond the practical aspects, emotional support is crucial:
   - **Active listening**: Being attentive to the person's feelings and concerns, without minimizing their emotions.
   - **Encouragement**: Reward effort and progress, however small, to boost self-confidence.
   - **Patience**: Respect the person's pace of learning and adaptation, without imposing excessive pressure.

Training methods

Relatives can be trained in a variety of ways to suit their availability and preferences:

- **Practical workshops**: Organized by associations or specialized centers, these sessions enable you to learn in real-life situations with experienced trainers.
- **Individual sessions**: A professional can come to your home for personalized training, taking into account your specific environment.
- **Online support**: Video tutorials, digital guides and webinars offer the flexibility to learn at your own pace.
- **Support groups**: Participating in groups with other relatives facing the same challenges provides an opportunity to exchange experiences and practical advice.

Involve the person concerned in the training

It is essential to consider the blind or partially-sighted person as a central player in his or her own life. Actively involving the person in the training of those close to him or her has several advantages:

- **Respect for autonomy**: Recognizing one's skills and preferences strengthens one's sense of control over one's life.
- **Personalization**: Each individual has unique needs and habits; his or her participation ensures that the training is adapted to his or her situation.
- **Strengthening relationships**: This collaboration fosters better mutual understanding and strengthens the relationship between the person and their loved ones.

Long-term benefits

Training relatives in assistance techniques has a lasting positive impact:

- **Improved quality of life**: adapted assistance promotes the independence and well-being of blind and partially-sighted people.
- **Reduced family stress**: Loved ones feel more confident and less anxious, knowing how to act effectively.
- **Accident prevention**: Better knowledge of guiding and safety techniques reduces the risk of falls or injury.
- **Social integration**: By facilitating participation in outside activities, training helps maintain an active social life.

Challenges to overcome

It is important to recognize that the training of relatives may encounter certain obstacles:

- **Availability**: Professional or personal constraints may limit the time loved ones can devote to training.
- **Resistance to change**: Some people may be reluctant to adopt new methods or technologies.
- **Emotional burden**: Accepting the situation and adapting to new responsibilities can be emotionally taxing.

To overcome these challenges, we recommend :

- **Training planning**: Organize sessions at appropriate times and define realistic objectives.
- **Encourage dialogue**: Encourage loved ones to express their feelings and share their concerns.
- **Seek support**: Call on professionals or peer groups for additional support.

Conflict management and family dynamics

- **Addressing disagreements about care**

The relationship between patients, their families and healthcare professionals is at the heart of effective, humane medical care.

However, disagreements sometimes arise about the care to be provided. These differences may concern diagnosis, treatment, care objectives or end-of-life decisions. Addressing these disagreements constructively is essential to preserving the quality of care, respecting patients' rights and maintaining a relationship of trust between all parties involved.

Understanding the origins of disagreements

Disagreements about care can arise for a variety of reasons, often linked to differences in perspective, values or understanding.

1. **Different perceptions and expectations**
   - **Patients and relatives**: They may have specific expectations based on their personal experiences, beliefs or the information they have gathered. They may want aggressive treatments to maximize the chances of recovery, or, on the contrary, prefer comfort and quality of life.
   - **Healthcare professionals**: Their approach is guided by medical knowledge, clinical protocols and experience. They can recommend treatments based on proven efficacy, risks and potential benefits.

2. **Communication barriers**
   - **Complex medical language**: The use of technical terms can lead to misunderstandings.
   - **Insufficient listening**: If the patient's concerns or questions are not fully heard, this can generate frustration.
   - **Cultural and linguistic differences**: These can affect the way information is perceived and interpreted.

3. **Personal values and beliefs**

    ○ **Religious or spiritual beliefs**: These can influence decisions about certain treatments, such as blood transfusions or surgery.
    ○ **Personal preferences**: Some patients may refuse invasive treatments or prefer alternative approaches.

The consequences of unresolved disagreements

Failure to deal effectively with disagreements can have significant negative repercussions:

- **Deterioration of the therapeutic relationship**: Trust between patient and caregiver may be compromised, affecting future cooperation.
- **Non-adherence to treatment**: A patient who disagrees is less likely to follow recommendations, which can compromise his or her recovery.
- **Increased stress**: Tensions can increase stress for all parties, including the family and care team.
- **Legal risks**: Unresolved disputes may lead to complaints or litigation.

Strategies for dealing with disagreements

1. **Open and empathetic communication**

    ○ **Active listening**: Taking the time to listen to the patient's concerns without interruption or judgment.
    ○ **Clarification**: Ask questions to make sure you understand the patient's point of view.
    ○ **Clear expression**: Explain medical information in accessible language, avoiding jargon.

2. **Sharing decisions**

    - **Involve the patient**: Encourage active participation in the decision-making process.
    - **Present the options**: Provide a complete description of the different possibilities, with their advantages and disadvantages.
    - **Respecting autonomy**: Recognizing patients' right to make decisions about their own health.

3. **Managing emotions**

    - **Recognize emotions**: Validate the patient's feelings, whether fear, anger or worry.
    - **Psychological support**: Offer the services of a psychologist or counselor if necessary.

4. **Mediation and third-party intervention**

    - **Involve neutral third parties**: A mediator, ethicist or other professional can help facilitate communication.
    - **Family meetings**: Organize family meetings to align expectations and concerns.

5. **Ongoing training for professionals**

    - **Developing communication skills**: Training in empathic communication and conflict management can improve caregivers' ability to deal with disagreements.
    - **Cultural awareness**: Understanding cultural influences can help you adapt your approach.

Ethical and legal considerations

1. **Respecting patient autonomy**

    ◦ **Informed consent**: Patients must be given all the information they need to make a free and informed decision.
    ◦ **Right of refusal**: A patient has the right to refuse treatment, even if the caregiver considers it to be against his or her best interests.

2. **Principle of beneficence and non-maleficence**

    ◦ **Acting in the patient's best interest**: Professionals must aim for the patient's best interests.
    ◦ **Avoid harm**: Do no harm to the patient, even in the event of disagreement.

3. **Confidentiality and privacy**

    ◦ **Protecting information** : Ensure the confidentiality of discussions and shared information.
    ◦ **Consent for sharing**: Obtain the patient's agreement before disclosing information to third parties.

The role of the care team

1. **Interdisciplinary work**

    ◦ **Collaboration between professionals**: Doctors, nurses, care assistants, psychologists and others need to work together to offer coherent care.
    ◦ **Information sharing**: Communicate effectively within the team to ensure that everyone is informed of disagreements and strategies in place.

2. **Support for caregivers**

    - **Supervision and debriefing**: Providing a space for caregivers to express their own frustrations or emotions linked to disagreements.
    - **Training and resources**: Provide the tools needed to manage difficult situations.

Preventing disagreements

1. **Establish a relationship of trust from the outset**

    - **Transparency**: Being honest about the uncertainties, risks and limitations of treatments.
    - **Availability**: Showing patients that they are supported and that their concerns are taken seriously.

2. **Patient education**

    - **Inform**: Provide appropriate educational resources to help patients understand their condition.
    - **Encourage questions**: Invite the patient to ask questions and express doubts.

3. **Cultural and personal preferences taken into account**

    - **Cultural adaptation**: Respect cultural practices and beliefs that may influence care decisions.
    - **Individualized care**: Avoiding standardized approaches and taking into account each patient's individual characteristics.

In the event of persistent disagreement

If, despite all efforts, the disagreement persists :

- **Documentation**: Record discussions, information provided and decisions made.
- **Referral to higher authorities**: Consult ethics committees or medical authorities for advice.
- **Respect the patient's choice**: As long as the patient's decisions do not endanger others, and as long as the patient is capable of making his or her own decisions, his or her choices must be respected.

- **Support for families in distress**

The family is the central nucleus of society, a place where every individual should find support, love and understanding. Yet some families face challenges that plunge them into deep distress. Whether financial difficulties, health problems, relationship conflicts or unexpected crises, these situations call for tailored support to help families overcome obstacles and regain balance. Supporting families in distress is therefore essential to preserve family cohesion, promote the well-being of each member and strengthen the social fabric as a whole.

Understanding family distress

Family distress can take many forms and stem from a variety of causes:

1. **Economic difficulties**: Job loss, over-indebtedness or insufficient income can generate significant stress, affecting family relationships and household stability.

2. **Health problems**: A chronic illness, disability or mental disorder affecting a family member can place a considerable emotional and financial burden on the whole household.

3. **Relationship conflicts**: Tensions between spouses, parents and children or siblings can erode communication and trust within the family.

4. **Traumatic events**: The death of a loved one, an accident, a natural disaster or any other disruptive event can profoundly destabilize family dynamics.

5. **Social isolation**: The lack of a support network, and geographical or cultural distance, can amplify feelings of loneliness and despair.

The importance of supporting families in distress

Supporting families in distress is crucial for several reasons:

- **Preventing problems from escalating**: Early intervention can prevent difficulties from escalating, thus avoiding more serious consequences such as family disintegration or psychological disorders.

- **Promoting mental and emotional well-being**: Adequate support helps family members manage stress, anxiety and depression, promoting better mental health.

- **Strengthening family ties**: By helping families to resolve their problems, we encourage communication, mutual understanding and solidarity.

- **Protecting children**: Children are particularly vulnerable to the effects of family distress. Appropriate support ensures their safety, development and education.

Available forms of support

1. **Psychological and therapeutic support**

    ○ **Family therapy**: aims to improve communication and resolve conflicts between family members, by working on relationship dynamics.

    ○ **Individual consultations**: enable each member to express their feelings, understand their emotions and develop strategies for coping with difficulties.

    ○ **Support groups**: provide a space for exchange with other families in similar situations, encouraging the sharing of experiences and solutions.

2. **Social and community support**

    ○ **Social services**: Social workers can assess the family's needs and offer financial, material or administrative assistance.

    ○ **Associations and non-governmental organizations**: They offer a variety of programs, workshops and activities designed to support families in difficulty.

    ○ **Community initiatives**: Community centers, churches or local groups can offer support, advice and resources.

3. **Financial and material support**

    ○ **Government assistance**: Family allowances, housing subsidies, healthcare or education grants can ease the financial burden.

- **Food banks and donations**: Provide food, clothing and other essential items to families in need.

- **Employment and training programs**: Help family members acquire new skills or find stable employment.

4. **Educational support**

    - **Parenting workshops and training**: Offer advice on parenting, stress management and child development.

    - **School support**: Tutoring or homework help programs for children, to prevent them from dropping out of school.

    - **Raising awareness of available resources**: Inform families about the services and assistance they can access.

The role of healthcare professionals and social workers

Health professionals, psychologists, counsellors and social workers play a key role in supporting families in distress:

- **Global assessment**: Identify the family's specific needs, whether emotional, financial or social.

- **Targeted intervention**: Suggest appropriate action plans, in collaboration with the family, to resolve identified problems.

- **Resource referral**: Direct families to appropriate services, whether financial assistance, therapy or community programs.

- **Ongoing monitoring**: Provide long-term support for the family's progress and adapt interventions if necessary.

Strategies for strengthening family support

1. **Developing support networks**

    - **Community mobilization**: Encouraging community participation to create a network of support for families in distress.
    - **Inter-institutional collaboration**: Promoting cooperation between different services (health, education, justice) for comprehensive care.

2. **Service accessibility**

    - **Simplifying procedures**: Reducing administrative hurdles to facilitate access to aid.
    - **Relocation of services**: Offer services directly in families' homes or in locations close to their homes.
    - **Adapted pricing**: Offer free or reduced-cost services for low-income families.

3. **Awareness-raising and information**

    - **Communication campaigns**: Informing the public about the signs of family distress and how to get help.
    - **Preventive education**: Integrate programs into schools or community centers to address

parenting skills, stress management and conflict resolution.

4. **Professional training**

    ○ **Skills development**: Provide ongoing training for caregivers on the most effective approaches to supporting families.

    ○ **Intercultural approach**: Training professionals in cultural diversity to better understand and respect families' values and traditions.

The importance of political and social commitment

Effective support for families in distress requires commitment at all levels:

- **Strong public policies**: Governments must invest in social services, mental health and family support programs.

- **Protective legislation**: Put in place laws that protect the rights of families, particularly in terms of housing, employment and health.

- **Collective responsibility**: Society as a whole must recognize the importance of supporting families in difficulty, by promoting solidarity and fighting stigmatization.

Encouraging family resilience

Resilience is a family's ability to face challenges, adapt and grow stronger despite difficulties. To foster this resilience :

- **Valuing strengths**: Recognizing and encouraging the family's internal skills and resources.

- **Promoting autonomy**: supporting families to become agents of their own change, by developing their self-confidence.

- **Creating positive links**: Strengthen relationships within the family and with the community to build a solid support network.

Chapter 10

Specific care in a variety of environments

Inpatient care

- **Specific protocols**

In the field of healthcare and assistance for people with disabilities, the establishment of and adherence to specific protocols are essential to guarantee high-quality, safe care tailored to individual needs. Specific protocols are detailed procedures that define the steps to be followed when carrying out a particular task or intervention. They serve as a guide for professionals, ensuring consistency of practice and contributing to the standardization of care, while enabling adaptation to the particularities of each patient.

Importance of specific protocols

1. **Patient and professional safety**

   Specific protocols are designed to minimize the risks associated with care. By clearly defining procedures, they reduce potential errors, omissions or misunderstandings. For blind or visually impaired patients, adapted protocols ensure their safety when moving around, undergoing medical procedures or using technological devices.

2. **Quality of care**

   By following proven protocols, healthcare professionals can offer high-quality care based on best practices and the latest scientific advances. This ensures that all patients receive optimal care, whatever the team or location.

3. **Consistency and continuity**

   Protocols promote a consistent approach between the various parties involved. This is particularly important when several professionals are involved in the care of the same patient. Consistent actions facilitate coordination and ensure continuity of care.

4. **Training and assessment**
   Protocols also serve as a basis for training new professionals and evaluating practices. They can be used to identify ongoing training needs and set up quality improvement programs.

Examples of specific protocols in the context of visual impairment

1. **Protocol for guiding blind or partially-sighted people**
   This protocol details the steps to follow when accompanying a visually-impaired person:
   - **Making contact**: Introduce yourself verbally, ask if the person would like help and obtain their consent before touching them.
   - **Positioning**: Offer your arm for the person to hold, moving slightly forward.
   - **Communication**: Describe the environment, point out obstacles, changes in terrain or direction.
   - **Overcoming obstacles**: Explain how to approach stairs, doorways or narrow passages, adapting your walking pace.

2. **Medication administration protocol for blind patients**
   This protocol is designed to ensure that patients take their medication correctly:
   - **Medication identification**: Use Braille labels, tactile color codes or compartmentalized boxes.
   - **Clear information**: verbally explain the drug's name, dosage, dosing schedule and possible side effects.
   - **Verification**: Confirm with the patient that he/she has understood the instructions and, if

possible, observe the medication being taken to ensure compliance with the prescription.

3. **Assistive technology protocol**
This protocol guides the patient in the learning and use of technological devices:

- **Needs assessment**: Identify the patient's specific needs in terms of communication, mobility or access to information.
- **Installation and configuration**: Ensure that devices are correctly installed and configured according to patient preferences (language, voice, volume).
- **Practical training**: Provide appropriate training, using suitable teaching methods and avoiding technical jargon.
- **Ongoing support**: offer assistance in the event of difficulties, and provide updates and additional training as required.

4. **Medical appointment management protocol for visually impaired patients**

- **Planning**: Suggest suitable schedules, taking into account the patient's mobility constraints.
- **Communication of information**: Provide appointment details (date, time, location) in an accessible format, e.g. audio or Braille.
- **Transportation and accompaniment**: If necessary, organize adapted transportation or accompaniment to the appointment.
- **On-site reception**: Provide a personalized welcome, guide patients around the premises and explain the consultation procedure.

5. **Therapeutic education protocol**
   This protocol aims to reinforce the patient's skills in managing his or her own health:

   ○ **Initial assessment**: Identify the patient's knowledge of his or her condition, needs and expectations.
   ○ **Learning objectives**: Define realistic and appropriate objectives, in collaboration with the patient.
   ○ **Teaching methods**: Use accessible media (audio, Braille, enlarged characters), individual or group sessions.
   ○ **Assessment**: Measure progress, adjust program if necessary, reward success.

Development and implementation of specific protocols

1. **Multidisciplinary participation**
   The development of protocols must involve a multidisciplinary team, including doctors, nurses, care assistants, occupational therapists, psychologists and, where appropriate, patient representatives. This collaboration ensures that protocols are complete, relevant and adapted to actual needs.

2. **Compliance with regulations and standards**
   Protocols must comply with current laws, regulations and recommendations. They must also incorporate good professional practice and recognized quality standards.

3. **Staff training**
   Adequate training is essential if staff are to apply protocols correctly. This includes initial and ongoing training sessions, practical workshops and regular skills assessments.

4. **Evaluation and continuous improvement**

    Protocols must be regularly reviewed and updated in line with feedback, scientific advances and changing patient needs. Evaluating their effectiveness enables us to identify strengths and areas for improvement.

Challenges and special considerations

1. **Personalized care**

    Although protocols provide a standardized framework, it is crucial to adapt them to the particularities of each patient. Professionals must be flexible and discerning in responding to individual needs, while respecting established procedures.

2. **Effective communication**

    Implementing protocols requires clear communication between members of the healthcare team and with the patient. It is important to use appropriate language, check understanding and encourage two-way communication.

3. **Resource management**

    The application of certain protocols may require additional resources in terms of time, personnel or equipment. It is important to plan and manage these resources to ensure the feasibility and sustainability of protocols.

4. **Cultural and ethical sensitivity**

    Protocols must take into account patients' cultural, ethical and religious considerations. Respect for diversity and consideration of individual preferences are essential for respectful and effective care.

- **Coordination with the medical team**

Coordination with the medical team is fundamental to ensuring optimal patient care. In healthcare, teamwork is essential to meet the complex and varied needs of individuals. Close collaboration between different professionals ensures continuity of care, improves the quality of interventions and promotes patient well-being. Understanding the importance of this coordination and implementing effective strategies to reinforce it is crucial in an increasingly complex medical environment.

The importance of interprofessional coordination

1. **Improved quality of care**
   Coordination between members of the medical team enables essential patient information to be shared, avoiding errors, redundancies or omissions in care. Fluid communication ensures that all professionals have the same data, facilitating informed, consistent decision-making.

2. **Continuity of care**
   Patients often interact with several healthcare professionals, such as doctors, nurses, care assistants, physiotherapists and other specialists. Effective coordination ensures that transitions between these different players run smoothly, ensuring uninterrupted, seamless care.

3. **Optimizing resources**
   By coordinating efforts, the medical team can use available resources more efficiently. This reduces waiting times, avoids redundant examinations or treatments, and concentrates efforts where they are most needed.

4. **Patient satisfaction**
   Good coordination contributes to strengthening patient

confidence in the healthcare system. Patients feel they are cared for holistically, their needs are better understood, and their concerns are addressed consistently by all professionals.

Key elements of successful coordination

1. **Effective communication**
   Communication is the cornerstone of coordination. It must be clear, concise and regular. Professionals must share relevant patient information, respecting confidentiality rules and using appropriate channels.

2. **Use of information technology**
   Electronic medical records, secure messaging systems and online collaboration platforms facilitate real-time information sharing. By adopting these tools, patient data can be centralized and made accessible to all team members.

3. **Interdisciplinary meetings**
   Regular meetings between the various professionals involved in patient care enable care plans to be discussed, challenges to be addressed and actions to be coordinated. These meetings also foster mutual understanding of each other's roles and competencies.

4. **Clarifying roles and responsibilities**
   It's essential that each team member knows exactly what his or her tasks are, and what the others' are. This avoids overlaps, gaps and misunderstandings. An organization chart or detailed care plan can help clarify these aspects.

5. **Training and professional development**
   Encouraging ongoing training and development of teamwork skills improves coordination. Professionals need to be trained in soft skills, such as interpersonal

communication, conflict resolution and collaborative leadership.

The challenges of coordination

1. **Communication barriers**
   Differences in terminology, staggered schedules and hierarchies can hamper communication. It's important to put strategies in place to overcome these barriers, such as establishing standardized communication protocols.

2. **High workload**
   Time and workload pressures can limit professionals' availability for coordination. It is crucial to recognize the importance of coordination and allocate time to it in schedules.

3. **Resistance to change**
   Some professionals may be reluctant to adopt new working methods or technologies. A participative approach, involving teams in the process of implementing change, can help reduce this resistance.

4. **Complex healthcare systems**
   Complex organizational structures, multiple levels of care and different policies can complicate coordination. A systemic approach, aimed at simplifying processes and harmonizing practices, is required.

Strategies for strengthening coordination

1. **Implementing standardized protocols**
   Developing clear protocols and procedures for routine processes can facilitate coordination. These protocols should be developed in collaboration with all team members, and regularly updated.

2. **Collaborative leadership**
   Leaders must encourage collaboration, value everyone's

contributions and promote a culture of teamwork. They play a key role in creating an environment where coordination is a priority.

3. **Patient involvement**
   Involving patients in their own care plan promotes coordination. The patient becomes an active member of the team, bringing a unique perspective on his or her needs and preferences.

4. **Evaluation and feedback**
   Putting in place mechanisms to evaluate the quality of coordination and gather feedback from professionals and patients helps identify areas for improvement and celebrate successes.

Care at home

- **Adapting the home environment**

The home environment is where we spend a large part of our lives, a place of comfort, safety and independence. For people who are blind or partially sighted, the home can present particular challenges that require specific adaptations. Adapting the home environment becomes an essential step in promoting independence, ensuring safety and improving quality of life. This adaptation is not limited to physical modifications, but encompasses a global approach that takes into account the individual needs, lifestyle habits and aspirations of each person.

The importance of home adaptation

Vision loss affects the way a person interacts with their environment. Visual cues, which are often taken for granted, become less reliable or non-existent, which can make daily tasks more complex and increase the risk of accidents. Adapting the home environment aims to compensate for these limitations by creating a functional, safe and comfortable space. It enables blind or partially-sighted people to maintain or regain their independence in activities of daily living, such as getting around, cooking, washing, dressing and managing the home.

Fundamental principles of adaptation

1. **Safety**
   Safety is the top priority when it comes to home design. The aim is to reduce the risk of falls, collisions or accidents in the home by eliminating obstacles, securing dangerous areas and facilitating circulation.

2. **Accessibility**
   Accessibility concerns the ease with which a person can reach, use and interact with the various elements of their environment. This means making objects, equipment and spaces usable without excessive effort or constant assistance.

3. **Simplicity and organization**
   A well-organized environment, where every object has its own place, helps reduce confusion and makes it easier to remember where things are. Simplicity in layout avoids unnecessary clutter and allows for better orientation.

4. **Personalization**
   Needs and preferences vary from person to person. It's essential to take into account lifestyle habits, degree of visual impairment and functional capabilities to adapt the environment appropriately.

Specific home improvements by zone

1. **Entrance and corridors**

    - **Clear passageways**: Corridors and entrances must be free of obstacles such as furniture, shoes or objects on the floor.
    - **Non-slip floor coverings**: Use non-slip mats or floor coverings to prevent falls.
    - **Suitable lighting**: For the visually impaired, sufficient glare-free lighting helps to distinguish passage areas.

2. **Lounge and living areas**

    - **Furniture layout**: Furniture should be arranged to create wide, unobstructed circulation spaces. Avoid furniture with protruding corners or low objects that are difficult to detect.
    - **Tactile cues**: Use different textures on furniture surfaces to facilitate identification by touch.
    - **Constant organization**: Maintain a fixed arrangement of furniture and objects to aid spatial memorization.

3. **Kitchen**

    - **Accessible equipment**: Install devices with tactile or voice controls, contrasting buttons or raised markings.
    - **Utensil organization**: Store kitchen utensils logically and consistently, by category and in specific locations.
    - **Safety**: Use induction hobs to reduce the risk of burns, and install automatic gas or electricity cut-offs.

- **Targeted lighting**: For the visually impaired, directed lighting on worktops helps to distinguish food and utensils.

4. **Bathroom**

    - **Non-slip coverings**: Install non-slip bath mats and safe floor coverings.
    - **Grab bars**: Place grab bars near bathtubs, showers and toilets to facilitate movement.
    - **Adapted taps**: Use single-lever or touch-sensing taps for ease of use.
    - **Visual contrasts**: For the visually impaired, use contrasting colors between equipment (washbasin, toilet) and walls to enhance perception.

5. **Bedroom**

    - **Functional layout**: position the bed so as to facilitate access to other areas of the room, such as the wardrobe or door.
    - **Organized storage**: Use modular storage systems with tactile or Braille labels to identify garments.
    - **Controlled lighting**: Install switches that are easily accessible from the bed, or use voice commands to control lighting.

6. **Stairs**

    - **Non-slip strips**: Install contrasting anti-slip strips on the steps to indicate the start and end of the staircase.
    - **Continuous handrail**: Install a solid handrail on each side of the staircase for additional support.
    - **Sufficient lighting**: Ensure uniform illumination with no annoying shadows or reflections.

Techniques and aids for adaptation

1. **Tactile markings**

    - **Embossed or Braille labels**: Use tactile labels to identify food products, medicines, documents or appliance controls.
    - **Tactile markings on appliances**: Place raised buttons on remote controls, keypads or household appliances to make them easier to use.

2. **Color contrasts**

    - **Use bright colors**: For the visually impaired, paint door frames, switches or handles in colors that contrast with the walls for better visibility.
    - **Crockery and utensils**: Choose crockery that contrasts with the table or worktop to distinguish between food and plates.

3. **Suitable lighting**

    - **Natural lighting**: Favor daylight, avoiding thick curtains that block light.
    - **Adjustable lamps**: Use lamps with flexible arms to direct light where it's needed.
    - **Avoid glare**: Install blinds or filters to reduce glare on shiny surfaces.

4. **Assistive technologies**

    - **Voice assistants**: use devices such as Alexa, Siri or Google Assistant to control lights, thermostats, alarms or get information.
    - **Talking devices**: Get watches, scales, thermometers or household appliances that provide voice guidance.

- **Mobile applications**: Use applications specially designed for the visually impaired, such as screen readers or object recognition software.

Tips for a successful adaptation

1. **Involving the person concerned**

    - **Active participation**: The blind or partially-sighted person must be at the heart of the adaptation process, expressing his or her needs, preferences and ideas.
    - **Personalization**: Adapting solutions to the individual's habits and lifestyle to ensure their relevance and effectiveness.

2. **Consult professionals**

    - **Occupational therapists**: These professionals can assess the home and suggest specific adaptations to improve functionality and safety.
    - **Locomotion instructors**: They can help develop techniques for getting around safely in the home and outdoors.
    - **Technical aids technicians**: They can recommend and install adapted technological devices.

3. **Evolving with the times**

    - **Regular reassessment**: Needs can change over time, so it's important to reassess the environment periodically to make adjustments.
    - **Technology updates**: Keep abreast of new technical aids or innovations that can improve quality of life.

Financial assistance and available resources

- **Subsidies and grants**: Financial aid may be available from government agencies, local authorities or associations to fund home improvements.
- **Specialized associations**: Organizations such as the Association Valentin Haüy or the Fédération des Aveugles de France offer advice, resources and sometimes financial support.
- **Tax credits**: Certain home adaptation expenses may be eligible for tax credits or deductions.

- **Planning visits and interventions**

Planning visits and interventions is a key element in the effective, personalized care of patients, particularly those with visual impairments. Careful organization of meetings between healthcare professionals, patients and their families ensures continuity of care, optimizes available resources and meets the specific needs of each individual. This includes coordinating the various players involved, adapting interventions to patients' schedules and rhythms, and putting in place strategies to anticipate and manage the unexpected.

The importance of planning in care

Careful planning of visits and interventions has several major advantages:

1. **Improved quality of care**: By organizing visits in a consistent way, healthcare professionals can devote the necessary time to each patient, ensuring complete, attentive care.

2. **Continuity of care**: Effective planning ensures that the various parties involved are informed of each other's actions, avoiding redundancies or omissions in the care provided.

3. **Respecting patient preferences**: By taking into account the patient's availability and preferences, planning promotes comfort and adherence to the care plan.

4. **Optimization of resources**: Precise organization enables efficient management of professional time and travel, reducing costs and waiting times.

Key steps in planning visits and interventions

1. **Initial needs assessment**
   The first step is to carry out a thorough assessment of the patient's needs. This includes:

   - **Medical analysis**: Understanding the patient's medical condition, treatment and follow-up requirements.
   - **Functional assessment**: Identify limitations related to visual impairment and the technical or human aids required.
   - **Psychosocial considerations**: Take into account the family context, available support and any barriers to care.

2. **Drawing up a personalized care plan**
   Based on the assessment, a care plan is drawn up in collaboration with the patient and, if necessary, his or her family. This plan must :

   - **Define objectives**: Clarify the goals to be achieved, whether medical, functional or psychological.
   - **Specify interventions**: Detail the actions to be carried out, the professionals involved and the frequency of visits.

- **Set a timetable**: Draw up a schedule of visits, taking into account the availability of both the patient and the caregivers.

3. **Coordination between professionals**
Collaboration between different members of the care team is essential. This involves :

    - **Regular communication**: Share relevant information via meetings, shared folders or secure communication tools.
    - **Role clarification**: Define responsibilities to avoid overlaps or gaps.
    - **Flexibility**: adapt the schedule to changes in the patient's condition or unforeseen events.

4. **Adapting to patient needs**
It's important to personalize visits so that they correspond as closely as possible to the patient's expectations and constraints:

    - **Appropriate schedules**: Offer slots that respect the patient's rhythm of life, avoiding uncomfortable or inappropriate times.
    - **Length of visit** : Allocate sufficient time to address all questions without rushing.
    - **Advance preparation**: Inform the patient in advance of the content of the visit so that he or she can prepare for it.

5. **Getting around**
For blind and partially-sighted patients, getting around can be a challenge:

    - **Home visits**: Whenever possible, we prefer to visit the patient's home to reduce the need for transport.

- **Organizing outside appointments**: If you need to go to the doctor's office or the hospital, you need to be accompanied or provided with suitable transportation.
- **Route optimization**: Group visits geographically to reduce travel time for professionals.

Using technology to facilitate planning

Technological tools can greatly improve planning efficiency:

1. **Care management software**
   - **Shared calendars**: Allows all participants to view schedules, coordinate visits and avoid scheduling conflicts.
   - **Alerts and reminders**: Send notifications to patients and professionals of upcoming appointments.

2. **Mobile applications for patients**
   - **Accessibility**: Applications adapted for the visually impaired, with voice interfaces or high contrast, make it easier to consult the schedule.
   - **Direct communication**: Enable patients to easily contact professionals, ask questions or report changes.

3. **Teleconsultations**
   - **Flexibility**: Remote consultations can complement face-to-face visits, offering a convenient alternative when travel is difficult.
   - **Regular follow-up**: maintain frequent contact with the patient to adjust care if necessary.

Anticipating and managing the unexpected

Despite careful planning, unforeseen events can occur:

1. **Emergency plans**

   - **Clear protocols**: Establish procedures for medical or social emergencies, with contacts to be reached and actions to be taken.
   - **Accessible information**: Patients and their families need to know about these protocols and how to react.

2. **Flexible planning**

   - **Reactivity**: Being able to quickly reorganize visits if necessary, whether to add a new service or postpone another.
   - **Effective communication**: Inform those concerned immediately of changes to avoid misunderstandings.

3. **Ongoing support**

   - **Available resources**: Provide patients with telephone numbers, support services or information on how to get help outside of scheduled visits.
   - **Proactive follow-up**: Professionals can take the initiative and contact the patient on a regular basis to make sure all is well.

Involving the patient in planning

The patient must be at the center of the planning process:

1. **Active participation**
    - **Consultation**: Ask for the patient's opinion on visiting times, frequency and schedule.
    - **Empowerment**: Encouraging patients to express their needs, preferences and concerns.

2. **Education**
    - **Clear information**: Explain the care plan, objectives and the role of each person involved to the patient.
    - **Training**: If the patient uses planning technologies, provide appropriate training so that he or she can use them independently.

3. **Respect and dignity**
    - **Personalization**: Recognize the uniqueness of each patient and adapt planning accordingly.
    - **Confidentiality**: Respect patient privacy in all communications and information exchanges.

Working with family members and caregivers

Relatives often play a crucial role in supporting the patient:

1. **Coordination**
    - **Involvement**: Include family members in the planning process if the patient wishes, taking into account their availability and ability to help.
    - **Communication**: Share relevant information with loved ones, while respecting the patient's wishes regarding confidentiality.

2. **Support for caregivers**

    ○ **Resources**: Provide caregivers with information and training so that they can support the patient effectively.
    ○ **Recognition**: Valuing the role of caregivers and offering them support to prevent burnout.

Assessment and adjustment of care plan

Planning is a dynamic process that must be regularly evaluated:

1. **Feedback**

    ○ **Gathering impressions** : Ask patients and professionals for their opinions on the course of visits and interventions.
    ○ **Feedback analysis**: Identify strengths and areas for improvement.

2. **Adjustments**

    ○ **Flexibility**: Modify the care plan according to the patient's changing condition, needs or preferences.
    ○ **Updating objectives**: Revise care plan objectives to keep them relevant and realistic.

3. **Quality of care**

    ○ **Indicators**: Use performance indicators to measure the effectiveness of planning (adherence to schedules, patient satisfaction, achievement of objectives).
    ○ **Continuous improvement**: Implement actions to constantly improve the quality of planning and care.

Rehabilitation centers and specialized institutions

- **Intensive rehabilitation programs**

Intensive rehabilitation is a therapeutic approach aimed at maximizing a person's functional capabilities following injury, illness or surgery. These programs are designed to speed up the recovery process, improve quality of life and encourage a return to independence. They are based on multi-disciplinary, personalized care tailored to the specific needs of each patient. At a time when medical advances are making it possible to treat complex pathologies more effectively, intensive rehabilitation is an essential complement to optimize clinical results.

Understanding intensive rehabilitation

Intensive rehabilitation is characterized by a high frequency of sessions, prolonged duration of interventions and increased intensity of exercises. Unlike traditional programs, which can be spread over a longer period with less frequent sessions, intensive rehabilitation concentrates efforts over a shorter period, with the aim of achieving significant progress in a shorter time.

This approach is particularly beneficial for patients with neurological, musculoskeletal or cardio-respiratory impairments. It also applies to people who have suffered head injuries, strokes, spinal cord injuries, or degenerative diseases such as multiple sclerosis or Parkinson's disease.

The fundamentals of intensive programs

1. **Individualized care**
   Every patient is unique, with individual needs, abilities and goals. Intensive rehabilitation programs are therefore tailor-made, following a thorough assessment of the patient's impairments, functional limitations and

aspirations. This personalization ensures that interventions are relevant and effective.

2. **Multidisciplinary approach**
Intensive rehabilitation mobilizes a team of healthcare professionals from different disciplines: rehabilitation physicians, physiotherapists, occupational therapists, speech therapists, neuropsychologists, nurses, dieticians and social workers. This inter-professional collaboration makes it possible to address all aspects of recovery, whether physical, cognitive, emotional or social.

3. **Active patient involvement**
The success of intensive rehabilitation depends on the active participation of the patient. Patients are encouraged to become fully involved in the program, to understand the objectives and to make the necessary efforts to achieve them. This involvement fosters motivation, adherence and autonomy.

4. **Use of advanced techniques and technologies**
Intensive programs often incorporate cutting-edge equipment and innovative methods: rehabilitation robots, exoskeletons, virtual reality, mirror therapy, functional electrical stimulation, biofeedback and more. These tools help intensify exercises, stimulate brain plasticity and promote functional recovery.

The benefits of intensive rehabilitation

1. **Improved functional capacity**
Frequent, intensive sessions speed up the recovery process. Patients can regain motor, cognitive and sensory functions more quickly, making it easier to return to daily, professional and social activities.

2. **Stimulation of neuroplasticity**
Intensive repetition of exercises promotes the reorganization of neural networks. The brain, capable of

adapting and compensating for damage, can thus develop new connections to restore lost or impaired functions.

3. **Reducing secondary complications**
   By regularly mobilizing patients, intensive rehabilitation helps prevent complications associated with prolonged immobility: muscle atrophy, joint stiffness, bedsores, circulatory or respiratory disorders.

4. **Positive psychological impact**
   The rapid progress observed thanks to the intensity of the program boosts patients' self-confidence and morale. The feeling of accomplishment and renewed hope are powerful motivators to continue efforts and commit fully to rehabilitation.

Examples of intensive rehabilitation programs

1. **Stroke rehabilitation**
   Stroke patients benefit greatly from intensive rehabilitation. Protocols include daily physiotherapy sessions to restore motor skills, occupational therapy to improve coordination and autonomy in activities of daily living, and speech therapy to restore communication and swallowing.

2. **Spinal cord injury programs**
   People with spinal cord injuries take part in intensive programs designed to maximize their functional potential. The use of exoskeletons or bodyweight-supported treadmills stimulates walking and strengthens muscles. Targeted therapies also help manage spasticity and neuropathic pain.

3. **Intensive cardiac rehabilitation**
   After a myocardial infarction or heart surgery, patients can take part in intensive cardiac rehabilitation programs. These combine supervised physical exercise,

education about risk factors, nutritional advice and psychological support. The aim is to reduce the risk of recurrence, improve physical capacity and promote a rapid return to activity.

4. **Programs for children with cerebral palsy**

   For children with cerebral palsy, intensive programs such as the Therasuit method or intensive motor therapy camps offer prolonged and repeated sessions over several weeks. These interventions aim to improve muscle tone, coordination and fine and gross motor skills.

The challenges and considerations of intensive rehabilitation

1. **Fatigue and overload**

   The intensity of the programs can lead to physical and mental fatigue in patients. It is crucial to adapt the pace and workload to individual capabilities, taking care to avoid overwork or demotivation.

2. **Accessibility and cost**

   Intensive programs require considerable human and material resources. The financial cost can be an obstacle for some patients, hence the importance of mobilizing insurance, public aid or associations to facilitate access to this care.

3. **Adherence to treatment**

   The success of the program depends on patient motivation. Professionals therefore need to create an encouraging environment, set realistic goals and offer ongoing support to maintain commitment.

4. **Interprofessional coordination**

   Collaboration between different professionals is essential, but can be complex to organize. Regular meetings, effective communication and a shared vision of objectives are necessary to ensure coherent care.

The role of family and friends

Family support plays a key role in the success of intensive rehabilitation programs. Relatives can encourage the patient, participate in certain sessions, help with home exercises and contribute to maintaining a positive environment. Their involvement promotes continuity of care and strengthens the patient's support network.

Future prospects for intensive rehabilitation

1. **Technological innovation**
   Advances in robotics, virtual reality and artificial intelligence are opening up new possibilities for intensifying and personalizing rehabilitation. These technologies make it possible to create stimulating environments, precisely measure progress and adapt exercises to the patient's needs in real time.

2. **Scientific research**
   Studies into brain plasticity, recovery mechanisms and the effectiveness of different rehabilitation methods are helping to refine protocols and develop approaches based on solid scientific evidence.

3. **Professional training**
   Therapists' specialization in intensive techniques and ongoing training are essential to guarantee quality care. The sharing of knowledge and best practices within the medical community encourages the evolution of rehabilitation standards.

4. **Integrating care into the community**
   The development of intensive rehabilitation programs in the outpatient or home setting extends access to care,

reduces costs and facilitates the social reintegration of patients.

Chapter 11

Legislation and rights for blind people

National and international legal framework

- **Accessibility and discrimination laws**

Accessibility and anti-discrimination laws are essential pillars in guaranteeing equal rights and opportunities for all citizens, especially for people with disabilities. They aim to ensure that everyone can participate fully in social, professional and cultural life, by removing physical, social and institutional barriers. These laws cover several key areas, including access to buildings, public services, employment, education and communication, while prohibiting all forms of discrimination based on disability. Their implementation is crucial to promoting an inclusive society that respects fundamental rights.

Context and international legal framework

The legal framework relating to accessibility and discrimination is part of an international drive to protect and promote the rights of people with disabilities. Reference texts include:

1. **The United Nations Convention on the Rights of Persons with Disabilities (CRPD)**
   Adopted in 2006, the CRPD is a fundamental international treaty that recognizes the rights of people with disabilities and requires member states to take measures to ensure their equality before the law. It stipulates that people with disabilities should be able to enjoy all human rights and fundamental freedoms without discrimination. The CRPD addresses key issues such as accessibility, social inclusion, education, employment and access to justice.

2. **Universal Declaration of Human Rights (1948)**
   Although the Declaration does not specifically mention disabled people, it enshrines the principles of freedom,

equality and non-discrimination, which apply to all people, regardless of their physical or mental condition.

Key aspects of accessibility legislation

1. **Accessibility of public and private spaces**
   Accessibility laws impose strict standards for the design of public buildings, private spaces accessible to the public (such as stores, hotels and restaurants), and transport infrastructures. These measures are designed to enable all people, especially those with physical or sensory limitations, to access these spaces freely and safely.

   - **Access ramp**: Wheelchair ramps are mandatory.
   - **Accessible elevators**: Installation of elevators in public and private buildings where stairs represent an obstacle.
   - **Adapted signage**: Use of Braille signs, pictograms or contrasting colors for the visually impaired.
   - **Adapted washrooms**: Toilets with sufficient space for wheelchair users, with grab bars and equipment at accessible height.

2. **Digital accessibility**
   In the digital age, accessibility also extends to information and communication technologies. Websites, mobile applications and interactive terminals must be designed to be usable by all, including the visually impaired, hearing impaired and those with cognitive disabilities.

   - **WCAG standards (Web Content Accessibility Guidelines)**: These international guidelines specify the criteria to be met to ensure that online content is accessible to all. They provide solutions such as compatibility with screen readers, subtitles for videos, and simplified navigation.

3. **Accessible public transport**
   Legislation requires public transport infrastructures (buses, trains, subways, planes) to be adapted to accommodate people with disabilities. This includes :

   - Accessible platforms and stops,
   - Reserved spaces in vehicles,
   - Visual and audible signals to inform people with hearing or visual impairments.

4. **Accessibility to health and education services**
   Health and education institutions are subject to accessibility standards to ensure that anyone, regardless of disability, can receive the care and instruction they need.

   - **Teaching aids**: Schools and universities have to make special arrangements to accommodate disabled students (course materials in Braille or digital format, support by specialized assistants, etc.).
   - **Access to care**: Healthcare facilities must be equipped to receive people with disabilities and provide them with quality care free of barriers related to their physical condition.

Fighting discrimination

Anti-discrimination laws aim to prevent and punish behavior or decisions based on prejudice against people with disabilities, in all aspects of public and private life. These laws apply to employment, education, access to services, and participation in social and political life.

1. **Direct and indirect discrimination**

    ◦ **Direct discrimination**: This occurs when disabled people are treated less favorably than others, because of their disability. For example, denying someone access to a job because of their physical disability.
    ◦ **Indirect discrimination**: This is more subtle, and occurs when seemingly neutral rules or practices have a disproportionate effect on disabled people. For example, requiring all job applicants to have perfect mobility for no justified reason.

2. **Equal employment opportunities**
The legislative framework requires employers to take steps to ensure equal opportunities in access to employment for people with disabilities. This includes:

    ◦ **Reasonable accommodation**: Adapting the workstation (flexible working hours, specific equipment) to enable the person to carry out his or her tasks.
    ◦ **Prohibition of discriminatory practices**: Recruiters must not exclude a candidate on the grounds of disability, unless this makes it objectively impossible to perform the essential tasks.

3. **Sanctions and remedies**
The law provides for penalties for acts of discrimination, whether at work, at school or in the community. Victims of discrimination can lodge complaints with the courts or with institutions specializing in the defense of human rights.

4. **Disability-related harassment**
Harassment, whether verbal, physical or moral, based

on disability is strictly forbidden. This includes mockery, intimidation or degrading behavior towards people with disabilities, whether at work, at school or in any other environment.

Implementation and monitoring of laws on accessibility and discrimination

For these laws to be effective, monitoring and control mechanisms need to be put in place. Governments, as well as local authorities, are responsible for ensuring that buildings, services and businesses comply with accessibility standards.

1. **Inspections and audits**: The authorities regularly inspect public places, businesses and services to check compliance with accessibility standards.

2. **Incentives and sanctions**: Governments may offer subsidies or financial aid to encourage companies to comply with accessibility laws. On the other hand, financial or legal sanctions may be imposed on offenders.

3. **Awareness-raising and training**: For accessibility and anti-discrimination laws to be fully effective, it is essential to raise awareness of the rights of people with disabilities among businesses, employers, healthcare and public service professionals, as well as the general population. Training programs on inclusion and accessibility must be set up at all levels.

Ongoing challenges and future prospects

Despite the progress made, challenges persist in implementing accessibility and anti-discrimination legislation. Many buildings, services and businesses are still not up to standard, due to high costs or a lack of awareness of legal obligations. In addition, discriminatory attitudes towards disabled people are still common in some sectors, demonstrating the need to step up awareness campaigns.

Future prospects include :

- **Strengthen enforcement**: Increase the number of inspections and toughen penalties for offenders.
- **Promote technological innovation**: Encourage the use of new technologies to improve accessibility, particularly in the digital and transport sectors.
- **Support community initiatives**: Involve disabled people's associations in the design and evaluation of public policies to ensure that their needs are taken into account.

- **International conventions (e.g. Convention on the Rights of Persons with Disabilities)**

International conventions play a crucial role in protecting and promoting the rights of people with disabilities worldwide. They establish universal standards and principles to ensure that people with disabilities enjoy the same rights and freedoms as all other citizens, without discrimination. Among these conventions, the **Convention on the Rights of Persons with Disabilities (CRPD)**, adopted by the United Nations General Assembly in 2006, is the most significant and most recent.

The CRPD, along with other relevant international conventions, represents a comprehensive legal and ethical framework aimed at strengthening the human rights, equality, inclusion and dignity of people with disabilities. It represents a major step forward for the rights of people with disabilities, moving away from a charitable and paternalistic vision to a human rights-based approach.

The Convention on the Rights of Persons with Disabilities (CRPD)

Adopted in 2006 and entered into force in 2008, the CRPD is a binding international treaty designed to ensure that people with disabilities can fully enjoy all human rights and fundamental freedoms. It is a legally binding convention, which means that states that have ratified it undertake to respect its provisions.

The CRPD is based on several fundamental principles:

1. **Respect for the intrinsic dignity, individual autonomy and independence** of people with disabilities.
2. **Non-discrimination**: Disabled people must enjoy the same rights as other citizens, without discrimination on the grounds of disability.
3. **Full and effective participation and inclusion in society**: Promoting the active participation of people with disabilities in all aspects of life, including decision-making that affects them.
4. **Respect for difference and acceptance of disabled people as part of human diversity and humanity**.
5. **Equal opportunities**: Ensuring that people with disabilities have equal access to services, employment, education, culture and all other aspects of life.
6. **Accessibility**: Making physical environments, information, communication and services accessible to people with disabilities.
7. **Equality between men and women**: Ensuring equal rights for men and women with disabilities.
8. **Respect for the development of disabled children's abilities** and their right to preserve their identity.

Main objectives of the CRPD

1. **Changing perceptions of disability**
    The CRPD marks an important transition from a medical approach to disability, where the disabled person is seen as someone to be "cured" or "cared for", to a human rights-based approach, which emphasizes the autonomy, dignity and equality of disabled people. It promotes the social model of disability, according to which environmental and social barriers are the main obstacles to the inclusion of people with disabilities.

2. **Promoting social inclusion**
    The CRPD emphasizes the participation of people with disabilities in society on an equal footing with others. This includes access to education, the labor market, health services, public infrastructure and culture, as well as the right to live independently and make their own decisions.

3. **Guaranteeing accessibility**
    One of the fundamental principles of the CRPD is to ensure that public infrastructures, services, information and communication are accessible to all. States Parties are required to take measures to make buildings, transport, information and communication technologies and other services accessible to people with disabilities.

4. **Protecting against discrimination and promoting equality**
    The Convention obliges States to adopt laws prohibiting discrimination on the grounds of disability in all areas of public and private life, including employment, education, social services and access to goods and services.

5. **Respecting the right to privacy and autonomy**
    The CRPD recognizes that people with disabilities have

the right to make their own decisions about their lives, including healthcare, financial management and social interactions. This includes respect for their privacy, as well as their right to safety and protection from exploitation and abuse.

Specific areas covered by the CRPD

1. **Civil and political rights**
   The CRPD guarantees that people with disabilities enjoy the same civil and political rights as all other citizens. This includes the right to vote, access to justice, protection from torture and ill-treatment, and protection from exploitation and abuse.

2. **Economic, social and cultural rights**
   The CRPD aims to ensure that people with disabilities can fully exercise their economic, social and cultural rights, such as access to education, employment, social security and a decent standard of living. States must also ensure that disabled people can participate in cultural, recreational and sporting life on an equal footing.

3. **Independent living and inclusion in the community**
   The Convention attaches great importance to the autonomy of people with disabilities. It recognizes their right to live independently and to choose their place of residence, as well as to have access to appropriate support services that enable them to participate fully in society.

4. **Inclusive education**
   One of the most innovative aspects of the CRPD is the recognition of the right of people with disabilities to inclusive education. This means that people with disabilities must have access to mainstream education, with the necessary accommodations and support to

enable them to learn under the same conditions as other students.

5. **Employment and work**
   The Convention stipulates that people with disabilities have the right to equal employment opportunities. States parties must take measures to promote the employment of people with disabilities, in particular by making workplaces accessible, prohibiting discrimination in hiring, and providing reasonable accommodation.

6. **Access to health care**
   The CRPD requires that people with disabilities have access to health services, including specialized care, on an equal footing with others. This includes the obligation for States to ensure that health services are accessible, without discrimination, and that health personnel are trained in the specific needs of people with disabilities.

CRPD monitoring mechanism

States that have ratified the CRPD are required to submit regular reports to the Committee on the Rights of Persons with Disabilities, an international body of experts charged with monitoring the implementation of the Convention. The Committee examines national reports and makes recommendations to help States improve their practices in the field of disability rights.

The Optional Protocol

In addition to the CRPD, an **Optional Protocol** allows individuals or groups to submit complaints directly to the Committee on the Rights of Persons with Disabilities when they believe their rights have been violated and all domestic remedies have been exhausted.

Other relevant international conventions

1. **Vienna Declaration (1993)**
   An outcome of the World Conference on Human Rights, the Vienna Declaration reaffirms the universal nature of human rights and emphasizes that the rights of disabled people must be fully respected within the framework of human rights.

2. **International Labor Organization (ILO) Convention** concerning Vocational Rehabilitation and Employment of Disabled Persons (1983)**
   This convention aims to promote equality of opportunity and treatment for disabled workers in employment, by encouraging member states to adopt policies and measures in favor of vocational integration.

Patient legal protection

- **Health rights**

Health rights are a fundamental aspect of human rights, guaranteeing every individual access to quality health care, protection of their physical and mental well-being, and informed decision-making about their own health. These rights are enshrined in a number of international conventions and national laws designed to protect human dignity, promote equity in access to healthcare and prohibit all forms of discrimination in the healthcare field. Recognition of these rights is essential to ensure that everyone can benefit from the best possible care, regardless of their socio-economic situation, origin or state of health.

The right to health: a global definition

The right to health is recognized as a fundamental human right by various international instruments. This right does not only mean access to medical care services, but encompasses a set of conditions that enable individuals to lead a healthy life.

Universal Declaration of Human Rights (1948)

Article 25 of the **Universal Declaration of Human Rights** establishes the right of everyone to a standard of living adequate for his or her health and well-being, including food, clothing, housing and medical care and necessary social services. It also includes the right to social security in the event of unemployment, sickness, disability or other circumstances beyond a person's control.

International Covenant on Economic, Social and Cultural Rights (ICESCR) (1966)

Article 12 of the **ICESCR** recognizes "the right of everyone to the enjoyment of the highest attainable standard of physical and mental health". This article is particularly important, as it obliges states to adopt measures to guarantee access to health care, prevent illness, improve working conditions, and combat inequalities in access to health services.

Convention on the Rights of Persons with Disabilities (2006)

Article 25 of the **Convention on the Rights of Persons with Disabilities (CRPD)** recognizes the right of persons with disabilities to "the enjoyment of the highest attainable standard of health without discrimination on the basis of disability". This text commits States to providing accessible health services, including disability-specific care, while guaranteeing the informed consent of the persons concerned.

Key health rights

Healthcare rights are vast, covering many aspects crucial to ensuring equitable access to care, as well as patient dignity and autonomy. Here are the main health-related rights:

1. **Right of access to healthcare**
   Every individual has the right to access essential health services without discrimination based on race, gender, social status, disability or any other distinction. This right also implies physical accessibility (of healthcare infrastructures), economic accessibility (affordable prices) and informational accessibility (access to information on care and treatment).

2. **The right to non-discrimination in care**
   Patients must be treated equally and with dignity, regardless of their gender, sexual orientation, disability, economic status or ethnic origin. Discrimination in access to healthcare is a violation of human rights and is expressly prohibited by instruments such as the Convention on the Rights of Persons with Disabilities and other international conventions.

3. **Right to information and informed consent**
   Patients have the right to receive clear, comprehensive and comprehensible information about their state of health, possible treatments and the associated risks and benefits. They also have the right to give or refuse informed consent to medical treatment. **Informed consent** is essential to respect patients' autonomy and dignity.

4. **Right to confidentiality and privacy**
   Confidentiality is a fundamental right in the relationship between patients and healthcare professionals. This means that all information concerning an individual's health must be treated with the utmost discretion. No

personal data may be shared without the patient's explicit consent, except in cases of emergency or when required by law.

5. **The right to quality care**
The right to health includes the right to quality care, which means that medical services must be safe, effective, based on scientific evidence, and provided by qualified professionals. This includes access to essential medicines, appropriate medical equipment, and health infrastructures adapted to patients' needs.

6. **Right to autonomy and self-determination**
Everyone has the right to make decisions about their own health, including the choice of treatment and the management of their health. This includes the right to refuse treatment or medical intervention, even if such refusal may affect one's health.

7. **The right to mental health**
The right to health is not limited to physical health. It also includes the right to mental health, which implies access to psychological and psychiatric care and appropriate social support. Mental health care must be accessible without stigma, and respect patients' dignity and autonomy.

8. **The right to palliative care**
People at the end of life or suffering from chronic illnesses have the right to palliative care, which aims to relieve pain and improve quality of life. This includes psychological, social and spiritual support, while respecting the patient's end-of-life wishes.

9. **The right to protection against disease and health risks**
States have an obligation to set up systems for preventing disease, monitoring health risks and

promoting public health. This includes the fight against epidemics, vaccination, health education, and the management of environmental factors that may affect the health of populations.

10. **Right to redress and recourse in the event of violation of health rights**
    If a patient's health rights are violated, whether through denial of care, negligence or discrimination, they have the right to seek redress through legal or administrative remedies. Healthcare systems and governments must put in place mechanisms that enable patients to lodge complaints and receive compensation in the event of harm.

Obligations of States and healthcare system players

Health-related rights are accompanied by obligations for governments and health system players, who must guarantee access to care and ensure that patients are protected. These obligations fall into three categories:

1. **Obligation to respect** : Governments must refrain from any action that would limit access to care or violate patients' rights. This includes respecting patients' autonomy and their right to refuse medical treatment.

2. **Obligation to protect**: Governments must protect citizens against any violation of their health rights, whether by private actors (e.g. insurance or pharmaceutical companies) or by third parties.

3. **Obligation to fulfil**: Governments must take steps to ensure equitable and universal access to healthcare, by developing infrastructure, training healthcare professionals, and ensuring the availability of essential medicines and services.

Specific rights for the disabled, children and the elderly

Certain vulnerable populations, such as the disabled, children and the elderly, benefit from specific health rights:

1. **People with disabilities**: The Convention on the Rights of Persons with Disabilities (CRPD) guarantees that people with disabilities have access to healthcare services of the same quality as everyone else. This includes care specific to their condition, as well as accommodations to meet their particular needs.

2. **Children** : The health rights of the child, enshrined in the Convention on the Rights of the Child (1989), guarantee that children have access to medical care, nutrition and living conditions conducive to their development. Children must receive medical care adapted to their age, and their right to information must be respected, taking into account their capacity to understand.

3. **Seniors**: Elderly people are entitled to care tailored to their specific needs, including geriatric services, palliative care and services to prevent age-related illnesses. Discrimination on the basis of age, including in access to health services, is prohibited.

Challenges and prospects

Despite the progress made in recognizing healthcare rights, many challenges remain, including inequalities in access to care, lack of resources in some countries, and discrimination based on origin, gender or disability. To improve access to healthcare, countries must continue to :

1. **Strengthen healthcare systems**: Improve infrastructures, train qualified professionals and guarantee the availability of essential drugs and equipment.

2. **Promoting equity**: Reducing inequalities between regions and social groups to ensure that everyone has access to the care they need, particularly in rural areas or disadvantaged neighborhoods.

3. **Adopt prevention policies**: Invest in disease prevention, notably through information campaigns, the promotion of healthy lifestyles, and the prevention of epidemics.

4. **Protect the rights of vulnerable populations**: Provide special protection for children, the elderly, people with disabilities and other vulnerable groups, ensuring they have access to the care they need.

- **Remedies for rights violations**

When health rights are violated, it is essential that individuals have recourse mechanisms to obtain justice and redress. Such violations may include denial of care, discrimination in access to health services, breaches of medical confidentiality, lack of information about treatment, or inappropriate treatment that causes harm. Remedies for violations of health rights vary according to legal systems and health structures, but they must be accessible, effective and guarantee fair redress.

Legal and administrative remedies

Legal and administrative remedies are one of the main ways in which people can defend their rights and challenge health-related violations. These mechanisms make it possible not only to punish those responsible, but also to prevent future violations by reinforcing the responsibility of healthcare players.

1. **Internal appeals within healthcare facilities**
   Many healthcare facilities have internal complaints mechanisms. Patients who feel their rights have been violated can lodge a complaint directly with the facility concerned, whether it's a hospital, clinic or health center. This process is generally less formal and quicker than legal recourse. Typical steps include:

   - **Filing a complaint**: The patient or his or her representative submits a written or oral complaint describing the violation of rights.
   - **Internal investigation**: The plant conducts an investigation to verify the facts and gather evidence.
   - **Decision**: If the complaint is found to be justified, the establishment may take corrective action (formal apology, financial compensation, improved practices, etc.).

2. **Recourse to health authorities and ombudsmen**
   In most countries, health authorities play a key role in the regulation and supervision of healthcare services. In the event of a rights violation, patients can turn to government health agencies or specialized ombudsmen for arbitration. These institutions can investigate complaints, impose sanctions on healthcare professionals or facilities, and recommend reforms.

   - **Inspecting health services**: These authorities can inspect hospitals, clinics and other facilities to ensure compliance with standards and patients' rights.
   - **Mediation**: A healthcare mediator or rights advocate can facilitate an amicable settlement between the patient and healthcare professionals,

enabling a rapid solution to be found without going to court.

3. **Legal recourse**
   If internal or administrative mechanisms fail, or if the violation is serious, patients can seek redress through the courts. Recourse to the courts ensures a thorough investigation and, in the event of proven responsibility, the imposition of legal sanctions.

   - **Civil claims**: Patients can take legal action to obtain compensation for medical negligence, discrimination, or violation of their rights (such as the right to information or informed consent). Financial compensation may be awarded in the event of physical or moral injury.
   - **Criminal proceedings**: In cases of serious violations, such as abuse, mistreatment or fraud, criminal proceedings can be brought against those responsible. This can result in fines, imprisonment or suspension of the right to practice for offending healthcare professionals.
   - **Administrative justice**: In some countries, the decisions of health authorities or public health establishments can be challenged before administrative courts, particularly when they infringe patients' rights.

4. **Human rights commissions and independent national bodies**
   Some countries have national human rights bodies or commissions for the protection of patients' rights, which can be called upon in the event of health-related rights violations. These commissions act as observers and guarantors of fundamental rights, and can issue recommendations or even sanctions.

5. **Professional orders**
   In many countries, healthcare professionals are regulated by professional orders (such as the Order of Physicians, Nurses or Pharmacists). These institutions have the power to deal with complaints of ethical violations or professional misconduct. Sanctions can include:

   - **Warning or reprimand**: In the event of minor misconduct, a moral sanction may be imposed on the healthcare professional.
   - **Suspension or striking off**: For more serious misconduct, the professional may be suspended or struck off, prohibiting him/her from exercising his/her profession for a specified period or permanently.

International appeals

When national remedies have been exhausted, or when national health systems do not effectively guarantee health rights, it is possible to appeal to international human rights bodies. These bodies can intervene in serious or systematic cases of rights violation, particularly in countries where domestic judicial mechanisms are lacking.

1. **United Nations Committee on Economic, Social and Cultural Rights**
   Article 12 of the **International Covenant on Economic, Social and Cultural Rights (ICESCR)** enshrines the right to health. Member states are required to submit regular reports on the implementation of health rights in their countries. In the event of serious violations, individuals or groups can submit complaints to the **Committee on Economic, Social and Cultural Rights**.

2. **European Court of Human Rights (ECHR)**
For European countries, the **European Court of Human Rights** is a major recourse in the event of violation of fundamental rights, including health rights. Patients can appeal to this court when they believe their country has violated articles of the European Convention on Human Rights, such as the right to life (article 2) or the prohibition of inhuman or degrading treatment (article 3), often linked to inadequate healthcare.

3. **Committee on the Rights of Persons with Disabilities (CRPD)**
The **Convention on the Rights of Persons with Disabilities** also offers a complaints mechanism via the **Committee on the Rights of Persons with Disabilities**. People with disabilities who feel that their rights have been violated in the field of health, for example due to denial of treatment, discrimination or lack of accessibility, can appeal to this Committee.

4. **Non-governmental organizations (NGOs)** and advocacy bodies
Numerous **international NGOs** and human rights organizations, such as **Human Rights Watch**, **Amnesty International** and **Médecins du Monde**, monitor and denounce violations of health-related rights. They can provide legal support, raise public awareness and put pressure on governments to reform their healthcare systems.

Compensation and redress

Redress mechanisms must not only guarantee recognition of violations, but also offer appropriate **reparation measures** for victims. These measures include :

1. **Financial compensation**: In the event of physical or moral injury, patients can obtain financial compensation to cover medical expenses, loss of income, physical damage and emotional suffering.

2. **Supplementary healthcare**: In some cases, compensation may take the form of free supplementary healthcare, such as corrective treatments, rehabilitative therapies or extended medical follow-up.

3. **Practice reform and sanctions**: Beyond individual compensation, structural reforms may be recommended to prevent repeat violations, such as changes in medical protocols, better training for healthcare professionals, or tighter regulation of healthcare facilities.

4. **Apologies and moral rehabilitation**: Healthcare establishments or professionals involved may be required to make an official apology to the victim, which constitutes a public acknowledgement of the error or fault committed.

Equitable access to remedies

For remedies to be truly effective, it is crucial to ensure that all people, including those from vulnerable groups, can access these mechanisms. This includes :

1. **Legal assistance**: Provide free or reduced-cost legal aid for people who cannot afford a lawyer. Patient associations or NGOs can also provide support in filing complaints and obtaining redress.

2. **Awareness**: Inform patients of their rights and the recourse mechanisms available to them through awareness campaigns and education programs in healthcare establishments.

3. **Accessibility of procedures**: Ensure that complaint procedures are accessible, particularly for people with disabilities, the blind or people with reading or writing difficulties.

The caregiver's role in advocacy

- **Patient awareness and education**

Patient awareness and education are essential components of modern healthcare, helping to improve autonomy, well-being and adherence to treatment. They aim to give patients the knowledge, skills and confidence to manage their health proactively. This approach is not limited to imparting information, but seeks to empower patients to become key players in the management of their own health, in collaboration with healthcare professionals.

The importance of patient awareness and education

1. **Improving autonomy**

    One of the main aims of patient education is to enhance autonomy. By being well-informed about their disease, treatments and options, patients can make informed decisions about their health. This includes making choices about treatments, managing symptoms and preventing complications. Autonomy helps reduce dependence on caregivers and improves self-confidence in managing one's condition.

2. **Adherence to treatment**

    Awareness plays a crucial role in treatment adherence. A patient who understands what is at stake in his or her treatment (the benefits, potential side effects and importance of regularity) is more likely to follow medical recommendations. This better understanding can reduce treatment dropouts and medication errors, which in turn improves clinical outcomes.

3. **Fewer complications and hospital admissions**
A well-informed patient is better able to identify early warning signs of complications or worsening of the disease. They will know when to consult a healthcare professional or adapt their treatment. This helps avoid unnecessary hospitalization and limit the progression of certain chronic conditions, such as diabetes, heart failure or hypertension.

4. **Improving the caregiver-patient relationship**
Patient education promotes a more balanced relationship between healthcare professional and patient, facilitating dialogue and collaboration. Patients are better informed, and feel more involved in the medical decisions that concern them. This creates a dynamic partnership, where care is no longer simply received, but co-constructed.

5. **Reducing health inequalities**
Awareness-raising and education can help reduce health inequalities, particularly among vulnerable populations who often have less access to information. By providing adapted and accessible educational resources, these groups can acquire the knowledge they need to better manage their health, regardless of their level of education or health skills.

Areas of patient education and awareness

1. **Understanding the disease**
A fundamental aspect of education is to help patients understand the nature of their disease, its causes,

symptoms, evolution and associated risk factors. For example, in the case of a chronic pathology such as diabetes, the patient needs to understand the role of glucose in the body, the effects of insulin, and the possible complications associated with poor glycemic management.

2. **Treatment management**
   Patients must be educated about their prescribed treatments, including medications, medical devices (such as insulin pumps or inhalers), and any surgical or therapeutic procedures. This includes information on :

   - Method of administration (oral, injection, etc.).
   - Schedules and dosage.
   - Possible side effects.
   - Drug interactions to avoid.
   - Common medication administration errors.

3. **Lifestyle modification and prevention**
   Prevention plays a crucial role in improving patient health and reducing risks. Patient education often includes advice on lifestyle habits to prevent complications, such as :

   - A balanced diet adapted to your condition.
   - Regular physical exercise.
   - Stress management and the importance of quality sleep.
   - Reducing or stopping smoking and alcohol consumption.

4. These recommendations must be personalized to meet the patient's specific needs, taking into account his or her preferences and abilities.

5. **Self-monitoring and symptom management**
   For certain chronic pathologies, self-monitoring is

crucial. Patients need to learn how to monitor their own health parameters, such as blood sugar levels for diabetics, blood pressure for hypertensives, or signs of respiratory disease exacerbation for asthmatics. They also need to know how to interpret these results, and when to adjust their treatment or consult a doctor.

6. **Patients' rights and responsibilities**
A sometimes overlooked aspect of education is informing patients of their rights, including the right to informed consent, confidentiality of medical information, and quality care. Patients also need to understand their responsibilities, including the importance of following medical recommendations, keeping appointments, and communicating honestly with healthcare professionals.

Methods and tools for patient awareness and education

1. **Individual consultations with healthcare professionals**
Doctors, nurses, pharmacists and other healthcare professionals play a central role in patient education. During consultations, they can explain the patient's condition, answer questions and help him or her understand prescribed treatments. These interactions must be open and adapted to the patient's level of understanding.

2. **Therapeutic education workshops**
Therapeutic education programs offer group or individual sessions to teach patients how to better manage their disease on a daily basis. These workshops cover topics such as managing diabetes, hypertension or chronic lung disease. They are led by qualified healthcare professionals and enable patients to exchange ideas with others facing similar challenges.

3. **Written and audiovisual media**
   Brochures, guides, videos and computer graphics are common tools used to inform patients. These materials must be accessible and easy to understand, avoiding medical jargon, and sometimes translated into different languages to adapt to the diversity of patients. They also enable patients to review information at their own pace.

4. **Mobile applications and digital tools**
   The development of information technologies has opened up new opportunities for patient education. Mobile health applications enable patients to track their health parameters, receive medication reminders and access educational resources. Some applications also offer teleconsultation functionalities or forums for exchanges with other patients and professionals.

5. **Support and self-help groups**
   Support groups enable patients to share their experiences, learn from others, and feel less isolated. These groups can be run by healthcare professionals or patient associations, and are particularly useful for those coping with chronic illnesses or difficult conditions, such as cancer or autoimmune diseases.

The challenges of patient education

1. **Comprehension and health skills**
   Not all patients have the same level of understanding of medical information. Some may have difficulty assimilating concepts related to their condition, which can limit their ability to follow recommendations. It is therefore important to adapt the level of discourse and use a variety of teaching methods to ensure that every patient can understand and apply the information received.

2. **Cultural and linguistic barriers**
   Cultural and linguistic differences can create barriers to communication between healthcare professionals and patients. It is essential to take these specificities into account and offer educational materials in different languages, while respecting cultural sensitivities.

3. **Limited access to information**
   In certain regions or for certain social groups, access to medical information may be limited. Patients may not have access to the necessary resources, whether for geographical, economic or technological reasons. It is crucial to implement strategies to reach these populations, notably through community services or homecare.

4. **Lack of time for healthcare professionals**
   Healthcare professionals, particularly in overloaded systems, sometimes have little time to explain treatments and care in detail to patients. This lack of time can lead to misunderstanding on the part of patients. It is therefore important to create spaces dedicated to therapeutic education, as a complement to medical consultations.

The importance of a personalized approach

Every patient has different education and awareness needs. One size does not fit all. Healthcare professionals should strive to personalize their advice and information materials according to the patient's individual characteristics, such as age, level of education, health skills, and social environment. Personalized education maximizes the chances of successful treatment adherence and optimal health management.

- **Reporting abuse**

Reporting abuse in the healthcare sector is crucial to protecting vulnerable patients and ensuring that their fundamental rights are respected. Abuse, whether physical, psychological, financial or medical, can have serious consequences for the health and well-being of the individuals concerned. Reporting mechanisms make it possible to denounce such violations, initiate procedures to protect victims, and prevent such acts from recurring. However, reporting abuse is a complex process, requiring greater awareness on the part of professionals, patients and their families.

Nature of abuse in the healthcare sector

Healthcare abuse can take many forms. Some are more visible, while others are more insidious. It can be committed by caregivers, family members, carers or healthcare institutions.

1. **Physical abuse**

    This type of abuse involves any form of bodily violence inflicted on a patient, whether in the form of blows, bruises, deprivation or unjustified physical restraint. In healthcare facilities, excessive use of force during treatment or unnecessary physical restraint, such as unjustified patient restraint, are common examples of physical abuse.

2. **Psychological and emotional abuse**

    Psychological abuse includes humiliation, threats, insults, or any form of verbal mistreatment that can lower the patient's self-esteem and harm his or her mental well-being. This can include neglecting the patient's emotional needs, depriving them of social interaction, or manipulating them through fear or guilt.

3. **Financial abuse**

    Financial abuse occurs when a patient's financial or

material resources are misappropriated by a caregiver, relative or carer. This can include stealing money, extorting money, or mismanaging the patient's bank accounts or assets, often without consent or by abusing the patient's trust.

4. **Medical abuse**
Medical abuses include treatments administered without the patient's informed consent, unwarranted or inappropriate interventions, or the over-prescription of drugs. It can also include medical negligence, when necessary care is deliberately omitted or delayed, leading to a deterioration in the patient's state of health.

5. **Neglect**
Neglect, although not always perceived as direct abuse, is a serious form of mistreatment. It is the refusal or omission to provide necessary care, whether medical, nutritional or psychological, and can occur in hospital or home settings. Neglect can result in injury, preventable illness or the deterioration of a patient's mental state.

Warning signs and abuse recognition

It is often difficult for victims to report abuse themselves, due to fear of reprisals, isolation, or a sense of shame. So it's crucial that healthcare professionals, caregivers and loved ones are alert to warning signs. Here are a few signs that may indicate abuse:

1. **Physical signs**: bruises, burns, unexplained fractures, signs of excessive restraint or malnutrition. These injuries may be concealed or inconsistently explained by caregivers or family members.

2. **Behavioural changes**: A patient who suddenly becomes anxious, depressed, distant or distrustful may be the

victim of emotional or psychological abuse. Withdrawal, irritability or irrational fear on the part of some people are indicators to be taken seriously.

3. **Financial problems**: unexplained disappearance of funds, or irregular bank transactions, may indicate financial abuse. A vulnerable patient may also be asked to sign legal documents without understanding their content.

4. **Deteriorating health without medical explanation**: If the patient's health deteriorates despite care, or if he or she shows signs of malnutrition, dehydration or lack of hygiene, this may be a sign of neglect.

5. **Social isolation**: A caregiver who prevents family visits or isolates the patient from social contacts may be trying to hide abuse. This isolation is often a means of controlling the victim and limiting his or her access to outside resources.

Mechanisms for reporting abuse

Reporting abuse is an essential process for protecting victims and ensuring that action is taken against perpetrators. There are several ways of reporting abuse, depending on the context and the seriousness of the incident.

1. **Internal reporting in healthcare facilities**
   In hospitals, nursing homes and other healthcare facilities, internal reporting procedures are often put in place to deal with cases of abuse. Caregivers, patients and family members can report abuse to designated officials, such as an **abuse referent** or **quality manager**. These reports may be anonymous and are then investigated internally.

2. **Reporting to health authorities**
   Health agencies and **medical and social services inspectors** can be notified in cases of abuse or neglect in a medical setting. These authorities have the power to investigate, sanction offending establishments or professionals, and take measures to protect victims.

3. **Reporting to law enforcement agencies**
   When abuse constitutes a criminal offence (such as physical violence, sexual abuse or theft), it must be reported to the police. **Local police, gendarmeries** or **units specializing** in the protection of vulnerable people are competent to receive such complaints. The victim or a relative can lodge a complaint directly, and a judicial investigation will be launched.

4. **Contacting professional associations**
   If the abuse is committed by a healthcare professional (doctor, nurse, orderly), it can be reported to the relevant **professional association** (such as the Ordre des Médecins or Ordre des Infirmiers). These orders have disciplinary committees that can punish offending members, ranging from a simple warning to striking off the roll.

5. **Hotlines and assistance services**
   Many countries have set up **toll-free numbers** or **hotlines** to report abuse, particularly for the elderly or people with disabilities. These services can collect testimonies confidentially and direct victims to the appropriate organizations for treatment.

6. **Reporting to rights protection associations**
   Patient rights associations and **anti-maltreatment organizations** also offer listening and counseling services. They support victims in their efforts, whether to file a complaint or seek protective solutions. These

associations can also raise awareness and advocate for the protection of vulnerable people.

Obstacles to reporting abuse

Reporting abuse, while crucial, comes up against a number of obstacles that complicate the process and often delay care for victims.

1. **Fear of reprisals**
   Victims of abuse, particularly in institutional or family contexts, may fear reprisals from the perpetrators. This fear can lead them to remain silent, for fear of making their situation worse, or of being further isolated or mistreated.

2. **Caregiver dependency**
   Many patients are in a situation of great dependence on their caregivers, whether family helpers or professionals. This relationship of dependence can create a dynamic of abuse of power, making it difficult for the victim to denounce the abuse or leave the situation.

3. **Lack of awareness**
   Many people, including the victims themselves, are not always aware that certain behaviors constitute abuse. Emotional abuse or neglect, for example, are often perceived as minor inconveniences rather than violations of rights.

4. **Social isolation**
   Victims of abuse, particularly the elderly or patients with disabilities, may suffer from social isolation that limits their ability to alert the authorities or seek help. Perpetrators may also seek to maintain this isolation in order to better control the victim.

5. **A complex process**
   Reporting procedures can be complex and intimidating for victims, especially those without family or legal support. The fear of having to testify, or of not being believed, is also a major obstacle to reporting abuse.

Measures to make it easier to report abuse

Several initiatives can be implemented to encourage reporting of abuse:

1. **Awareness-raising campaigns**: It is essential to raise awareness among the general public, patients, families and healthcare professionals of abuse and the importance of reporting it. Communication campaigns can help disseminate information on reporting mechanisms and patients' rights.

2. **Professional training**: Caregivers need to be trained to identify signs of abuse and be aware of reporting procedures. This includes better training in patient rights, ethics and victim support.

3. **Simplified procedures**: Reporting mechanisms must be accessible and simple to use. Complaints must be confidential and anonymous if necessary, and victims must be supported throughout the process.

4. **Whistleblower protection**: It is important to protect those who report abuse, whether they are victims themselves, relatives or healthcare professionals. Laws must ensure that blowers-whistle are not subjected to reprisals.

Chapter 12

Complementary and alternative approaches

Sensory therapies

- **Music therapy**

Music therapy is a therapeutic discipline that uses music-sound, rhythm, melody and harmony-to promote the mental, physical and emotional health of individuals. For people who are blind or visually impaired, music therapy offers specific benefits by exploiting their heightened auditory sensitivity and providing a powerful means of expression and communication. It contributes to greater autonomy, self-confidence and social integration, while helping to overcome the challenges associated with vision loss.

The importance of music therapy for blind people

1. **Stimulation of the remaining senses**

   Sight deprivation often leads to compensation through the other senses, particularly hearing. Music therapy exploits this heightened auditory sensitivity to stimulate cognitive, emotional and motor skills. Music thus becomes an essential tool for exploring the environment, understanding the world and interacting with others.

2. **Emotional expression and communication**

   Music offers a universal language that transcends visual barriers. For blind people, it enables complex emotions to be expressed without the need for visual aids. Music therapy also facilitates communication with therapists and loved ones, providing a non-verbal means of sharing feelings and thoughts.

3. **Developing motor and sensory skills**

   Playing an instrument or participating in rhythmic activities can improve coordination, fine motor skills and tactile perception. These skills are crucial for blind people, as they contribute to greater independence in daily activities.

4. **Boosting self-confidence and self-esteem**
Successful musical training can have a positive impact on self-esteem. By taking on challenges and acquiring new skills, blind people develop self-confidence that is reflected in other aspects of their lives.

5. **Social integration and interaction**
Participation in music groups or music therapy workshops promotes social interaction. Music creates a common ground where blind people can connect with others, share experiences and feel part of a community.

Specific music therapy techniques for the blind

1. **Musical improvisation**
Improvisation encourages spontaneous expression and creativity. Music therapists can use easy-to-handle instruments, such as percussion, to allow patients to freely explore sounds and rhythms.

2. **Active and receptive listening**
Listening to different pieces of music helps evoke emotions, memories and mental images. This technique can induce states of deep relaxation or stimulate imagination and reflection.

3. **Singing and vocalization**
Using the voice as an instrument is particularly beneficial for blind people. Singing strengthens breathing, improves articulation and enables direct emotional expression.

4. **Rhythmic games and movement**
Combining music with physical movement helps develop body awareness and coordination. Rhythmic activities can include simple dance steps or body percussion.

5. **Use of appropriate technologies**
   Accessible electronic instruments and music creation software open up new possibilities. Devices with tactile feedback or voice synthesizers enable blind people to compose and perform music independently.

Therapeutic benefits observed

- **Improving cognitive functions**
  Music therapy stimulates memory, attention and learning skills. It can help develop strategies to compensate for the challenges associated with blindness.

- **Managing emotions and stress**
  Music has the power to regulate emotions, helping to reduce anxiety, depression or frustration often associated with vision loss.

- **Developing social skills**
  Group musical activities encourage cooperation, mutual listening and communication, strengthening social bonds and a sense of belonging.

- **Promoting independence**
  By strengthening motor and cognitive skills, music therapy contributes to greater independence in daily life.

Training music therapists to work with the blind

It is essential that music therapists are specially trained to meet the needs of blind people. This means:

- **Understanding specific challenges**
  Knowing the impact of blindness on emotional, social and cognitive development enables us to adapt interventions appropriately.

- **Appropriate communication**
 Use detailed verbal descriptions, pay attention to auditory and tactile cues, and encourage open, empathetic communication.

- **Designing the environment**
 Create a safe, accessible space, avoiding obstacles and ensuring that instruments are arranged logically and coherently.

- **Cultural awareness**
 Respect each individual's cultural and personal background, integrating musical styles that are familiar and meaningful to them.

Case studies and research

Research has demonstrated the effectiveness of music therapy with blind children, particularly in language development, improved social skills and sensory stimulation. In adults, music therapy has been associated with better psychological adaptation, reduced feelings of isolation and improved quality of life.

For example, music therapy programs in schools have shown that blind children attending regular sessions developed greater self-confidence and were more socially engaged. Similarly, in rehabilitation centers, blind adults have benefited from music therapy to manage the stress associated with vision loss and to redefine their personal identity.

Practical applications and recommendations

- **Integration into educational programs**
 Include music therapy in special schools and inclusive education programs to support the overall development of blind children.

- **Family support**
  Involving families in the therapeutic process can strengthen emotional bonds and provide additional support for the patient.

- **Interdisciplinary collaboration**
  Work as a team with other healthcare professionals-psychologists, occupational therapists, special educators-to create comprehensive intervention plans.

- **Accessibility of services**
  Promote access to music therapy for blind people by developing community programs and raising public awareness of the benefits of this approach.

- **Aromatherapy**

Aromatherapy is a discipline that uses essential oils extracted from aromatic plants to promote physical, emotional and mental well-being. For people who are blind or visually impaired, aromatherapy offers an enriching sensory dimension, by stimulating the sense of smell, a sense they often lack. This holistic approach can help improve quality of life, providing relaxation, soothing or revitalizing benefits, depending on individual needs.

The importance of the sense of smell for blind people

Loss of vision often leads to compensation through the other senses, notably smell. Blind people develop heightened olfactory sensitivity, enabling them to perceive finer nuances of scent and to navigate their environment using olfactory cues. Aromatherapy takes advantage of this sensitivity to offer rich and beneficial sensory experiences.

Benefits of aromatherapy for the blind

1. **Managing stress and anxiety**
   Essential oils such as lavender, chamomile or ylang-ylang are renowned for their soothing properties. Diffusing them can help reduce stress, anxiety or nervous tension, promoting a state of relaxation and well-being.

2. **Improved sleep**
   Sleep disorders are common among blind people, due to circadian rhythm disturbances linked to the absence of light perception. Essential oils such as lavender or marjoram can help you fall asleep and improve the quality of your sleep.

3. **Cognitive stimulation**
   Certain essential oils, such as rosemary or lemon, have stimulating properties that can help improve concentration, memory and alertness. They can be useful for activities requiring special attention.

4. **Emotional balance**
   Essential oils act on the limbic system, the region of the brain involved in emotions. Fragrances such as rose, neroli or jasmine can help regulate moods, bring comfort or stimulate positive feelings.

5. **Enhancing sensory autonomy**
   Aromatherapy enables blind people to further develop their olfactory sense, by exploring a variety of scents and learning to recognize them. This enhances their ability to interact with the environment and find their way around using olfactory cues.

Aromatherapy application techniques

1. **Atmospheric diffusion**
   The use of essential oil diffusers enables aromas to be

dispersed in the ambient air. It's a simple, safe way to benefit from the properties of essential oils, whether at home, in health centers or relaxation areas.

2. **Direct inhalation**
Inhaling from a handkerchief impregnated with a few drops of essential oil, or using personal inhalers, can offer a rapid effect, particularly for managing stress or moments of anxiety.

3. **Aromatic massages**
Massages with essential oils diluted in vegetable oil combine the benefits of touch and olfaction. For blind people, aromatic massage can be a complete sensory experience, promoting muscular relaxation and emotional balance.

4. **Aromatic baths**
Adding a few drops of essential oil diluted in a dispersant to bath water can provide a moment of deep relaxation. Aromatic baths combine the benefits of hot water and aromas to soothe body and mind.

Precautions for use

It is important to take certain precautions when using essential oils:

- **Proper dilution**: Essential oils are highly concentrated and must be diluted before application to the skin to avoid irritation or allergic reactions.

- **Choosing essential oils**: Some oils are not recommended for certain people (pregnant women, children, people with specific health problems). It is advisable to consult an aromatherapy professional for personalized advice.

- **Tolerance test**: Before using for the first time, perform a test by applying a small amount of the preparation to the inside of the wrist to check for any skin reaction.

- **Avoid contact with mucous membranes**: Essential oils must not come into contact with eyes, ears or mucous membranes.

Integrating aromatherapy into everyday life

1. **Creating a personalized olfactory ambience**
   Blind people can choose essential oils according to their olfactory preferences and current needs. Creating a customized olfactory ambience promotes a pleasant, reassuring environment.

2. **Olfactory workshops**
   By taking part in introductory workshops on essential oils, you can discover a variety of fragrances and learn to recognize and combine them. These workshops can be organized by aromatherapy professionals, and are an opportunity for exchange and sharing.

3. **Use in therapeutic support**
   Aromatherapy can complement other therapeutic approaches, such as music therapy, meditation or yoga. It enriches the sensory experience and can reinforce the beneficial effects of these practices.

The role of aromatherapy professionals

Aromatherapists are trained to advise and support people in the use of essential oils. They can :

- **Assessing individual needs**: Taking into account the person's state of health, preferences and goals.

- **Suggest appropriate synergies**: Combine several essential oils for optimum effect.

- **Inform about precautions**: Provide recommendations for safe and effective use.

- **Follow-up**: Adapt advice according to the person's changing needs and feelings.

Adapted physical activities

- **Yoga and meditation**

Yoga and meditation are age-old practices that promote harmony between body and mind. For people who are blind or visually impaired, these disciplines offer unique benefits, helping to strengthen body awareness, emotional balance and overall well-being. The absence of vision is not an obstacle to the practice of yoga and meditation; on the contrary, it can enrich the experience by focusing attention on internal sensations and the perception of movement.

The importance of yoga for blind people

1. **Developing body awareness**
   Yoga emphasizes the connection between body and mind. For blind people, this practice helps to refine the perception of movements, positions and body alignment. In the absence of visual cues, attention is focused on internal sensations, strengthening proprioception-awareness of the position and movement of different parts of the body.

2. **Improving balance and coordination**
   Yoga asanas (postures) require balance and coordination. For blind people, working on these aspects contributes to greater stability in daily movements, reducing the risk of falls and boosting self-confidence during physical activities.

3. **Managing stress and emotions**
   Yoga includes breathing (pranayama) and relaxation

techniques that help reduce stress, anxiety and mental fatigue. Regular practice promotes a state of inner calm and better emotional management, which is beneficial for psychological well-being.

4. **Muscle strengthening and flexibility**
Yoga postures stretch and tone muscles, improving strength, flexibility and posture. This is particularly important for blind people, who may adopt compensatory positions or experience muscle tension due to the use of a cane or guide dog.

Adapting yoga for the blind

Practicing yoga for blind people requires some adaptations to ensure a safe and beneficial experience:

1. **Detailed verbal guidance**
Instructors should provide clear, precise verbal descriptions of the postures, indicating the movements to be performed, the alignments to be respected and the sensations to be sought. It's important to use simple language, avoiding technical jargon, and to break down the postures step by step.

2. **Using touch**
With the participant's consent, the teacher may use tactile adjustments to correct alignments or help understand posture. Tactile indications should be gentle and respectful, taking care to ensure the practitioner's comfort.

3. **Safe environment**
The practice room must be laid out in such a way as to avoid obstacles and potential hazards. Mats must be

well positioned, and the space around the practitioner must be clear to allow safe movement.

4. **Adapting postures**
Certain postures can be modified or replaced to suit the abilities and comfort of the blind practitioner. Emphasis can be placed on simple, accessible postures, avoiding positions that could cause excessive loss of balance.

Recommended yoga techniques

1. **Simple standing postures**
Asanas such as mountain (Tadasana), tree (Vrikshasana) or warrior (Virabhadrasana) help to work on balance and leg strength. These postures reinforce stability and confidence in the standing posture.

2. **Seated and floor postures**
Seated postures, such as the easy posture (Sukhasana) or the butterfly posture (Baddha Konasana), are ideal for focusing on breathing and flexibility. Floor postures, such as cobra (Bhujangasana) or child (Balasana), offer stretching and relaxation.

3. **Breathing practices (Pranayama)**
Breathing exercises such as abdominal breathing, alternate breathing (Nadi Shodhana) or full breathing are essential for developing breath awareness, calming the mind and increasing vital energy.

4. **Relaxation and guided meditation**
Deep relaxation sessions, such as yoga nidra, and guided meditations help release physical and mental tensions, promoting a state of deep relaxation and clarity of mind.

Meditation for the blind

Meditation is a universal practice that does not depend on vision. It offers blind people a powerful means of developing concentration, managing stress and cultivating inner peace.

1. **Focus on the inner senses**
   In the absence of visual stimuli, the other senses become more predominant. Meditation can focus on bodily sensations, surrounding sounds or breathing, enabling deep immersion in the present experience.

2. **Adapted meditation techniques**

   ○ **Mindfulness meditation**: Paying non-judgmental attention to the sensations of the present moment, be they sounds, smells, tactile sensations or thoughts that arise.

   ○ **Inner visualization**: Although the person can't see, they can create mental images or internal feelings, such as imagining a soothing light or energy flowing through the body.

   ○ **Sound meditation**: Focus on sounds, whether environmental (birdsong, nature sounds) or musical (Tibetan bowls, mantras), to enter a meditative state.

3. **Specific benefits**
   Meditation helps to develop resilience in the face of daily challenges, reduce anxiety and improve mood. It also promotes better management of chronic pain or physical discomfort.

The role of instructors and specialized centers

1. **Teacher training**
   Yoga and meditation instructors need to be sensitized to

the specific needs of blind people. Specialized training is recommended to acquire the necessary skills in verbal communication, tactile adjustments and adapting practices.

2. **Inclusive yoga centers**
   Some centers or associations offer yoga classes adapted for blind people, providing a welcoming and suitable environment. These spaces also encourage meetings and sharing between participants.

3. **Use of adapted media**
   Audio recordings, accessible mobile applications or Braille guides can help practitioners to continue practicing independently at home.

Testimonials and feedback

Many blind people who have integrated yoga and meditation into their daily lives testify to the benefits they have experienced:

- **Improved mobility and balance**: greater ease of movement, straighter posture and reduced muscle tension.

- **Emotional management**: A greater ability to cope with stress, frustration and the challenges of blindness.

- **Strengthening social ties**: Taking part in yoga classes offers opportunities to meet other people, share experiences and break isolation.

- **Sports for the blind (goalball, judo)**

Sport is essential to the physical and psychological well-being of every individual. For blind and partially-sighted people, sport offers not only the usual benefits of physical activity, but also unique opportunities for personal development, social integration and self-improvement. Among the disciplines adapted for the visually impaired, **goalball** and **judo** take pride of place. These sports are specifically designed or adapted to enable blind athletes to achieve their full potential, exploiting their abilities and overcoming the challenges associated with sight loss.

The importance of sport for blind people

Sport plays a crucial role in the lives of blind people for several reasons:

1. **Improved physical condition**: Sporting activity strengthens muscles, improves endurance and promotes motor coordination, all of which are essential for daily independence.

2. **Building self-confidence**: Taking part in sporting activities provides an opportunity to meet challenges, boosting self-esteem and a positive perception of one's own abilities.

3. **Social integration**: Sport is an effective way of meeting other people, forging links and fostering inclusion within the community.

4. **Stress management and mental well-being**: Exercise releases endorphins, helping to reduce anxiety and depression and improve overall mood.

Goalball: a sport specially designed for the blind

Origin and history of goalball

Goalball was created in 1946 by Austrian Hanz Lorenzen and German Sepp Reindle, with the aim of rehabilitating World War II veterans who had lost their sight. Introduced to the Paralympic Games in 1976, it is now played all over the world and is one of the few sports designed exclusively for blind and partially-sighted people.

Game principles and rules

Goalball pits two teams of three players against each other on a rectangular pitch 18 meters long and 9 meters wide. Each end of the field has a goal that extends across the entire width.

- **Sound ball**: The ball used has bells inside, enabling players to locate it by hearing.

- **Silence required**: During the game, silence is maintained in the audience and by non-active players to allow better auditory perception.

- **Opaque masks**: All players wear opaque masks to equalize vision levels, ensuring fairness between participants.

- **Objective of the game**: Throw the ball by hand towards the opponent's goal while defending your own goal by blocking the ball with your body.

Goalball benefits blind players

- **Improved auditory acuity**: Sport develops the ability to detect and locate sounds accurately.

- **Development of coordination and mobility**: Quick movements and defensive actions improve flexibility and reactivity.

- **Team spirit and communication**: Goalball strengthens cohesion between players, requiring effective communication and mutual trust.

- **Competition and achievement**: Offering competitive opportunities at different levels, goalball enables athletes to set goals and celebrate their successes.

Accessibility and promotion of goalball

Many countries have national federations that promote goalball. Local clubs offer training and introductory courses for all ages. The sport also features in international competitions, such as the World Championships and the Paralympic Games, under the aegis of the International Blind Sports Federation (IBSA).

Adapted judo for the blind

Judo, an inclusive martial art

Judo, a Japanese martial art founded by Jigoro Kano in 1882, is based on the principles of flexibility, respect and maximum efficiency with minimum effort. It has been adapted for blind and visually impaired judokas, enabling these athletes to practice the sport safely and competitively. Judo for the visually impaired has been included in the Paralympic Games since 1988 for men and 2004 for women.

Specific judo adaptations for the blind

- **Initial contact**: Fights start with both judokas in physical contact, holding the opponent's judogi, to compensate for the absence of visual cues.

- **Adapted refereeing**: Referees use clear verbal signals to indicate actions, fight stoppages and mat exits.

- **Safe fighting surface**: Measures are taken to guarantee the safety of athletes, notably by adapting surfaces and increasing vigilance in the event of a fall.

The benefits of judo for blind people

- **Physical strengthening**: Judo develops strength, endurance, flexibility and balance.

- **Spatial and tactile perception**: gripping and throwing techniques improve body awareness and perception of the opponent's movements.

- **Discipline and respect**: Judo instills values of respect, self-control and perseverance.

- **Self-confidence**: Mastering techniques and taking part in competitions boosts self-esteem and self-confidence.

Integration into clubs and competitions

Many judo clubs welcome blind people, often in collaboration with specialized associations. Coaches receive training to adapt their teaching. Blind judokas take part in national and international competitions, offering opportunities for high-level sport.

Other adapted sports for blind people

In addition to goalball and judo, a variety of sports are accessible to blind people:

- **Athletics**: Guide races, long jump, shot put.
- **Swimming**: Adapted with tactile signals to indicate turns.
- **5-a-side soccer**: Football with a sound ball and adapted rules.
- **Tandem cycling**: a sighted rider guides the blind cyclist.
- **Skiing**: Downhill and cross-country skiing with voice guides.
- **Horseback riding**: Therapeutic or sporting, promoting balance and confidence.
- **Climbing**: with verbal instructions and appropriate safety equipment.
- **Rowing**: Crewed with sighted or blind teammates.

Initiatives and programs to promote sport

- **Specialized associations**: Organizations such as the Association Valentin Haüy and the Fédération Française Handisport offer resources, training and events to encourage the practice of sport.
- **Sports events**: National and international competitions, such as the Paralympic Games, highlight the achievements of blind athletes.

- **Educational programs**: Integrating adapted sports into schools and specialized institutions to encourage practice from an early age.

- **Awareness-raising and funding**: Campaigns to raise public and sponsor awareness of the importance of sport for blind people, helping to fund adapted equipment and infrastructure.

Challenges and prospects

Despite progress, challenges remain:

- **Accessibility**: Adapted and accessible infrastructures for regular practice.

- **Coach training**: More coaches need to be trained in the specificities of visual impairment.

- **Raising public awareness**: Combating prejudice and promoting a positive image of blind athletes.

- **Funding**: Find resources to support clubs, competitions and athletes, especially those aiming for the top level.

Future prospects are promising, with growing interest in adapted sports and increased recognition of the achievements of blind athletes.

Art and creative expression

- **Plastic art workshops**

Art is a universal language that transcends the barriers of verbal and visual communication. For people who are blind or visually impaired, access to visual art offers a unique opportunity for expression, creativity and connection with the world around them. **Plastic art workshops for the blind** are designed to harness the remaining senses, particularly touch, to enable these individuals to participate fully in artistic activities. These workshops are not only spaces for creation, but also for personal development, socialization and discovery.

The importance of art for blind people

1. **Personal expression and creativity**

   Art offers a means of expressing emotions, thoughts and experiences that may be difficult to verbalize. For blind people, plastic art enables them to materialize their inner world using tactile materials. Artistic creation becomes a vehicle for freedom and autonomy, where imagination knows no bounds.

2. **Sensory stimulation**

   Art workshops stimulate the senses of touch, hearing and sometimes even smell. The different textures, shapes and materials used enrich the sensory experience, contributing to the development of tactile and haptic abilities, which can enhance interaction with the everyday environment.

3. **Social integration**

   Taking part in group workshops encourages encounters with other people who share the same interests. This helps break the isolation often associated with blindness, forging links and developing a sense of belonging to an artistic community.

4. **Boosting self-esteem**
   Completing a work of art brings a sense of accomplishment and pride. Positive feedback from peers, instructors and the public boosts self-confidence and recognition of one's own talents.

Teaching approaches and techniques

1. **Adapting teaching methods**
   Specialized instructors develop adapted teaching methods, focusing on tactile and auditory sensations. Verbal explanations are detailed, and demonstrations can be carried out by guiding participants' hands to help them feel the gestures and techniques.

2. **Use of tactile materials**

    - **Clay and modeling clay**: These malleable materials can be used to create three-dimensional sculptures, encouraging the exploration of shapes and volumes.
    - **Textiles and fibers**: Weaving, embroidery or knitting offer rich tactile experiences, with a variety of textures.
    - **Natural materials**: Wood, stone, sand or shells bring different sensations and stimulate creativity.
    - **Relief painting**: using thick paints or gels to create two-dimensional works with palpable reliefs.

3. **Specific techniques**

    - **Tactile sculpture**: Encourage participants to model shapes based on their tactile perception, without visual reference.

- **Relief painting**: Use stencils, adhesives or relief materials to create images that can be felt by touch.
- **Tactile collage**: Assemble different materials on a surface to create textured compositions.
- **Braille drawings**: Integrate Braille into artwork to add a narrative or descriptive dimension.

4. **Technology integration**

    - **3D printing**: enable participants to design virtual objects that can then be materialized in three dimensions.
    - **Haptic devices**: Using technological tools that translate visual information into tactile sensations.

Role of instructors and reception structures

1. **Specialized training for instructors**
   Teachers need to be trained in the specifics of art education for blind people. This includes a thorough understanding of sensory needs, adapted techniques and inclusive teaching approaches.

2. **Creating a safe, accessible environment**
   Workshops must be designed to ensure the safety of participants, with clear spaces, safe tools and logical organization of materials. Movement must be facilitated, and potential hazards eliminated.

3. **Encouragement and recognition**
   Instructors play a crucial role in keeping participants motivated. They must encourage exploration, value efforts and celebrate achievements, while offering personalized support.

Examples of successful workshops and initiatives

1. **Accessible museums**
   Some museums offer tactile workshops, where blind visitors can touch reproductions of works of art, or even originals, for a complete artistic experience. Sensory itineraries are also set up to discover art through touch, hearing and smell.

2. **Educational programs**
   Specialized schools and centers are integrating visual art into their programs, recognizing its importance for the overall development of blind students. These initiatives promote inclusion and equal opportunities.

3. **Associations and art groups**
   Associations dedicated to art for blind people regularly organize workshops, exhibitions and events to promote the talents of these artists and raise public awareness.

Benefits observed in participants

1. **Development of motor skills**
   Handling artistic materials improves manual dexterity, coordination and precision of movement, which can have a positive impact on everyday activities.

2. **Cultural and intellectual enrichment**
   Art is a gateway to culture, history and ideas. Workshops provide an opportunity for learning and exchange, stimulating curiosity and critical thinking.

3. **Strengthening emotional well-being**
   Artistic creation is therapeutic. It helps to externalize emotions, manage stress and find inner balance.

Challenges and prospects

1. **Accessibility and financing**
   The development of specialized workshops requires financial resources for the purchase of adapted materials, instructor training and space planning. It is essential to mobilize public and private support to ensure the sustainability of these initiatives.

2. **Awareness and recognition**
   It's important to raise public awareness of the artistic abilities of blind people. This involves organizing exhibitions, taking part in cultural events and promoting the works produced.

3. **Pedagogical innovation**
   Continuing to innovate in teaching methods and technologies will expand the opportunities available to participants. The integration of new technologies, such as haptic virtual reality, could open up new perspectives.

- **Theater and oral expression**

Theater and oral expression offer a unique space for creativity, communication and personal development. For people who are blind or partially sighted, these artistic disciplines represent not only a source of artistic fulfillment, but also a powerful means of boosting self-confidence, autonomy and social integration. Blindness is not an obstacle in the world of theater; on the contrary, it can enrich the stage experience by emphasizing voice, body language and active listening.

The importance of theater for blind people

1. **Self-expression and creativity**
   Theater enables people to express their emotions, ideas and imagination freely and creatively. For blind people, the stage becomes a space where they can explore different characters, situations and feelings, without the limitations that society might impose on them.

2. **Building self-confidence**
   Taking part in theatrical activities helps to develop self-confidence. By taking up the challenge of performing in front of an audience, blind actors overcome fears and apprehensions, resulting in greater self-confidence in everyday life.

3. **Improving communication skills**
   Theater focuses on voice, diction, intonation and verbal expression. By working on these aspects, blind people improve their ability to communicate effectively, which is essential for social and professional interaction.

4. **Developing active listening and sensory perception**
   The absence of vision accentuates the importance of the other senses. Theater helps to refine listening skills and perception of sounds, silences and intonation, as well as sensitivity to the vibrations and movements of stage partners.

5. **Social integration and teamwork**
   Theater is a collaborative activity requiring cooperation between actors, directors and technical staff. Theatrical workshops provide an environment conducive to encounters, exchanges and the development of interpersonal relationships.

Adapted teaching approaches and techniques

1. **Auditory and verbal memory**
   Blind actors develop a remarkable auditory memory, which helps them retain texts, stage directions and their partners' lines. Rehearsals are based on careful listening and oral rehearsal.

2. **Tactile space setting**
   Tactile exploration of the stage allows actors to find their way around the scenic space. Raised floor markings and tactile or audible cues can be used to facilitate safe movement.

3. **Bodywork and movement**
   Body language is essential to theater. Workshops focus on body awareness, posture, gesture and movement. Specific exercises help actors express emotions and intentions through the body.

4. **Exploiting the voice**
   The voice is a major instrument for blind actors. Working on projection, modulation, rhythm and articulation enriches oral expression and brings characters to life.

5. **Use of assistive technologies**
   Tools such as audio recordings, accessible mobile apps or tactile feedback devices can help with learning scripts, staging and rehearsal coordination.

Examples of theatrical practice for the blind

1. **Improv workshops**
   Theatrical improvisation encourages spontaneity, creativity and adaptation. It enables actors to react in real time to their partners' proposals, relying on listening and intuition.

2. **Sensory theater**
   This type of theater focuses on sensations, sounds, smells and textures. Shows can be designed to be perceived without sight, involving the audience in an immersive experience.

3. **Dramatized readings**
   Aloud readings of plays offer an alternative way of concentrating on the text and vocal interpretation, without the need for complex stage movements.

4. **Collective creation**
   Collaborative writing and directing allow blind actors to actively participate in the design of the show, contributing their ideas and shaping characters and situations according to their experiences.

The role of directors and trainers

1. **Awareness-raising and specific training**
   Theater professionals need to be trained to work with blind actors, understanding their needs and adapting teaching methods. This includes clear communication, patience and encouragement.

2. **Adapting work methods**
   Stage directors can use detailed verbal descriptions, tactile demonstrations and adapted exercises to convey stage instructions.

3. **Creating an inclusive environment**
   It's essential to foster a climate of trust and respect, where every participant feels valued and supported. Including blind people in mixed troupes can enrich artistic work and promote diversity.

Benefits observed in participants

1. **Improving mobility and orientation**
   Theatrical practice helps develop skills for moving around in space, improving independence in daily life.

2. **Development of social skills**
   Working in a group encourages communication, active listening and empathy, strengthening interpersonal relations.

3. **Reducing isolation**
   Taking part in cultural and artistic activities helps to break down social isolation, offering opportunities for encounters and exchanges.

4. **Expressing and managing emotions**
   Theater offers an outlet for expressing deep feelings, managing stress and developing a better understanding of oneself.

Notable initiatives and programs

1. **Specialized theater companies**
   A number of theater companies are dedicated to blind or partially-sighted actors, offering original and innovative shows. These companies play a crucial role in promoting cultural accessibility.

2. **Workshops in schools and associations**
   Educational programs include theater for young blind people, fostering their personal development from an early age.

3. **Festivals and cultural events**
   Specialized festivals and inclusive programs showcase the work of blind artists, raising public awareness of their talent and creativity.

Challenges and prospects

1. **Accessibility and funding**
   Developing theatrical programs for blind people requires financial and logistical resources. It is important to mobilize public and private support to ensure the continuity of these initiatives.

2. **Raising public awareness**
   It is essential to change perceptions and stereotypes about the abilities of blind people. Broadcasting shows and publicizing artistic successes help to raise awareness.

3. **Professional training**
   Reinforce the training of directors, teachers and specialized educators so that they are better equipped to work with blind actors.

Chapter 13

Emergency preparedness

Appropriate first aid

- **Basic techniques**

First aid is a set of simple but essential gestures that can save lives in the event of an accident or illness. When it comes to people with specific needs, such as the disabled, it is crucial to adapt these techniques to ensure effective and respectful assistance. Adapted first aid aims to take into account the physical, sensory or cognitive particularities of victims, in order to provide appropriate assistance while preserving their dignity and comfort.

Understanding the importance of appropriate first aid

The aim of first aid is to stabilize the victim's condition until professional help arrives. In the case of people with special needs, an adapted approach is required to :

- **Ensuring the safety of the victim and the rescuer**: It's important to be aware of the person's particular characteristics to avoid any inappropriate or dangerous gestures.
- **Communicating effectively** : Adapt your communication to be understood and reassure the victim.
- **Provide appropriate assistance**: Adapt first aid techniques to the person's abilities and limitations.

General principles of adapted first aid

1. **Assessing the situation**
   Before intervening, it's essential to quickly assess the situation to identify potential hazards and understand the victim's specific needs.
   - **Safety**: Make sure the environment is safe to avoid endangering yourself or making the situation worse.

- **Observation**: Note visible signs of distress, technical aids (wheelchair, white cane) or behaviors that indicate an invisible disability.

2. **Approaching the victim**
    - **Introduction**: Introduce yourself calmly, stating your name and role, e.g. "Hello, my name is [Name], I'm trained in first aid, can I help you?"
    - **Consent**: Ask permission to help, except in a life-threatening emergency where the victim is unconscious.
    - **Adapted communication**: Use clear language, avoid medical jargon, and adapt communication (gestures, words, visual aids) to the person's abilities.

3. **Respect and dignity**
    - **Empathy**: Show understanding and patience.
    - **Autonomy**: Encourage the victim to take part in first aid if he/she can.
    - **Confidentiality**: Respect the individual's privacy, especially in the presence of others.

Basic techniques adapted to specific needs

1. **People with reduced mobility**
    - **Transfers and travel**
        - **Avoid moving the victim** unless there is imminent danger.
        - **Using technical aids**: If the person is in a wheelchair, ask if they prefer to sit or lie down.

- **Safe lifting techniques**: If moving is necessary, use appropriate techniques to avoid injury.
- **Lateral safety position (PLS)**
  - **Adaptation**: If the victim is unable to move to the side due to joint stiffness, keep the head tilted to the side to open the airway.

2. **Hearing-impaired and deaf people**
   - **Communication**
     - **Face to face**: Stand in front of the victim so that he or she can read lips.
     - **Articulation**: Speak clearly, without shouting or exaggerating mouth movements.
     - **Visual aids**: Use gestures, writing or pictograms if necessary.
   - **Visual signals**
     - **Universal gestures**: Learning a few basic signs can facilitate communication (for example, the sign for "pain" or "help").

3. **Visually impaired or blind people**
   - **Verbal presentation**
     - **Describe actions**: Explain each gesture before carrying it out.
     - **Guiding**: Offer your arm to guide the person if they need to move.
     - **Clarity**: Avoid expressions like "over here" or "over there", preferring precise indications ("two steps to the left").

4. **People with cognitive or intellectual disabilities**

    ○ **Language simplification**

    - **Short messages**: Use simple, direct sentences.
    - **Repetition**: Do not hesitate to repeat or reformulate if necessary.
    - **Patience**: Give the person time to understand and respond.

    ○ **Calming and reassuring**

    - **Soothing attitude**: Speak softly, avoid sudden gestures.
    - **Avoid over-stimulation**: Reduce noise and distractions.

5. **People with autism spectrum disorders**

    ○ **Respect for personal space**

    - **Avoid unnecessary physical contact**: Some people may be sensitive to touch.
    - **Announce gestures**: Explain what you're going to do before you do it.

    ○ **Direct communication**

    - **Clear instructions**: use concrete language and avoid metaphors.
    - **Observe reactions**: Watch for signs of stress or anxiety.

Specific first aid techniques

1. **Cardiorespiratory arrest**

    ○ **Cardiopulmonary resuscitation (CPR)**
    - **Adaptation**: For wheelchair users, if wheelchair extraction is not possible,

perform chest compressions with the patient seated, stabilizing the back.
- **Automatic external defibrillator (AED)**: Make sure electrodes are correctly positioned, taking into account physical particularities.

2. **Airway obstruction**

    - **Clearance techniques**
        - **Back slap**: Apply between the shoulder blades, in a position adapted to the person's mobility.
        - **Abdominal compression (Heimlich maneuver)**: For wheelchair users, kneel behind the patient to perform the maneuver.

3. **External bleeding**

    - **Direct compression**
        - **Wound access**: Ask permission before uncovering the wounded area.
        - **Maintaining pressure**: If possible, let the person apply pressure to the wound themselves.

4. **Discomfort**

    - **Diabetes**
        - **Recognize the signs**: confusion, paleness, sweating.
        - **Action**: If the person is conscious and can swallow, give them a source of quick sugar (sugar drink, glucose).

- Epilepsy
    - **Do not impede movement**: Protect yourself from injury by keeping dangerous objects out of the way.
    - **After the seizure**: Place the person in the lateral position and monitor breathing.

5. Burns
    - Cooling
        - **Temperate water**: Cool the affected area under water for at least 10 minutes.
        - **Beware of sensitivities**: Some people may have reduced sensitivity, so monitor water temperature to avoid hypothermia.

Calling for help

- **Key information to be provided**
    - **Precise location**: exact address, landmarks.
    - **Nature of emergency**: Clearly describe the situation and the victim's specific needs.
    - **State of consciousness**: Indicate whether the person is conscious, breathing, bleeding, etc.
    - **Special features**: Mention disability or special needs so that emergency services can be prepared.

Tips for first-aiders

1. **Continuing education**
    - **Regular training**: Participate in specialized first aid training.
    - **Updates** : Keep abreast of new techniques and protocols.

2. **Empathy and respect**
    - **Active listening**: Take the victim's suggestions on how best to help into account.
    - **Avoid prejudice**: Don't make assumptions about the person's abilities.

3. **Working with professionals**
    - **Relay with emergency services**: Pass on all information gathered to professionals on their arrival.
    - **Observation**: Note any changes in the victim's condition while waiting.

- **Crisis communication**

please develop in a fluid style and as little fragmented as possible:

Evacuation and safety plans

- **Adapting emergency protocols**

Adapting emergency protocols is essential to ensure the safety and well-being of all people in critical situations, especially those with disabilities. Traditional emergency protocols, often designed for the general population, may not take into account the specific needs of the blind or visually impaired, people with reduced mobility, or those with cognitive or sensory disabilities. It is therefore essential to review and modify these protocols so that they are inclusive, effective and provide equitable protection for all.

The importance of an inclusive approach

Emergencies, whether fires, natural disasters, terrorist attacks or other crises, demand a rapid, coordinated response. An inclusive approach means that everyone, regardless of ability, has access to the information and resources they need to protect themselves. This means:

1. **Accessible information**: Evacuation instructions and warnings must be available in a variety of forms, such as audible messages for blind people, clear visual signals for deaf people, and simple, comprehensible messages for those with cognitive impairments.

2. **Staff training**: Emergency responders, including firefighters, security guards and medical personnel, must be trained to understand the specific needs of people with disabilities and how to assist them effectively.

3. **Adapted infrastructure**: Buildings and public spaces must be designed or modified to facilitate evacuation for people with reduced mobility, with ramps, emergency elevators and accessible emergency exits.

Key elements for adapting emergency protocols

1. **Assessing specific needs**
   It is essential to understand the specific needs of the population concerned. This can be achieved by :
   - Conducting building accessibility audits.
   - Consulting people with disabilities and the organizations that represent them.
   - Identifying potential obstacles in current procedures.

2. **Effective communication**

    - **Multiple alert systems**: Use audible alarms, light signals, vibrations or text messages to reach all individuals.
    - **Clear, concise messages**: Instructions should be easy to understand, avoiding technical jargon.
    - **Inclusive language**: Adapting language to make it accessible to those with comprehension difficulties.

3. **Training and awareness-raising**

    - **Trained personnel**: Train employees and emergency personnel on how to assist people with disabilities.
    - **Inclusive emergency simulations**: Organize evacuation exercises that include people with disabilities to test and improve protocols.
    - **Public awareness**: Inform the entire community about what to do in the event of an emergency, with an emphasis on mutual aid and inclusion.

4. **Physical improvements**

    - **Accessible escape routes**: Ensure that escape routes are clear, wide enough and equipped to accommodate wheelchairs or people with mobility aids.
    - **Adapted signage**: Install Braille signs, tactile floor markings and color contrasts to help the visually impaired.
    - **Areas of refuge**: Provide safe spaces where people who can't use the stairs can wait for help.

5. Assistive technologies

   - **Emergency mobile applications**: Develop accessible applications that provide real-time alerts and instructions.
   - **Locating devices**: Use GPS technologies to help locate people in distress.
   - **Real-time information systems**: Set up platforms that disseminate up-to-date information accessible to all.

The specific case of blind or partially sighted people

For blind and partially sighted people, certain adaptations are particularly important:

- **Auditory guidance**: Use clear voice prompts to direct people to emergency exits.
- **Audible beacons**: Install devices that emit specific sounds to indicate directions or exit locations.
- **Human accompaniment**: Train staff and other occupants to assist blind people by guiding them appropriately.
- **Tactile equipment**: Use relief maps or tactile models to familiarize blind people with locations and evacuation routes during training sessions.

Integrating people with disabilities into emergency planning

Involving people with disabilities in the planning process is crucial to ensuring that protocols really do meet their needs. This can be achieved by :

- **Regular consultation**: Organize meetings with representatives of the disabled to gather their suggestions and concerns.

- **Participation in drills**: Invite people with disabilities to actively participate in emergency simulations to test the effectiveness of adaptations.
- **Ongoing evaluation**: Put in place mechanisms to gather feedback after each exercise or real-life emergency situation, in order to constantly improve protocols.

Collaboration with specialist organizations

Working with associations and accessibility experts can help develop innovative and effective solutions. These organizations can provide :

- **Technical expertise**: Advice on best practices in accessibility and communication.
- **Educational resources**: Training materials for staff and the public.
- **Support during operations**: Assistance in emergency situations thanks to their knowledge of specific needs.

Examples of best practice

- **Installation of evacuation ramps**: In some buildings, ramps have been installed to enable wheelchair users to descend stairs in complete safety.
- **Adapted warning systems**: Some cities have installed alarm sirens with multilingual voice messages and light signals to reach as many people as possible.
- **Braille evacuation maps**: Some establishments offer tactile maps to help blind people familiarize themselves with the premises.
- **Dedicated assistance team**: Training of volunteers or staff members specifically responsible for assisting disabled people in the event of an emergency.

Challenges and possible solutions

1. **Lack of resources**
   - **Solution**: Seek public or private funding, establish partnerships with non-governmental organizations, and integrate accessibility into project design to reduce long-term costs.
2. **Resistance to change**
   - **Solution**: Raise awareness of the importance of inclusion, present concrete cases where adaptations have saved lives, and encourage a culture of solidarity and respect.
3. **Complexity of requirements**
   - **Solution**: Adopt a personalized approach, recognizing that each individual has unique needs, and encourage flexibility in protocols to adapt to different situations.

- **Training for exceptional situations (fires, natural disasters)**

Exceptional situations, such as fires and natural disasters, represent major challenges for public safety. Emergency training is essential to prepare individuals and communities to respond effectively to these unpredictable events. Proper preparation can save lives, reduce property damage and facilitate recovery after a crisis. This training must be inclusive, taking into account the specific needs of each individual, including those with disabilities, to ensure a coordinated and effective response.

The importance of training for exceptional situations

1. **Preventing and minimizing risks**
   Knowledge of emergency procedures helps prevent accidents and minimize risks during a crisis. An informed population is better able to make rapid, appropriate decisions, thereby reducing potential consequences.

2. **Building community resilience**
   Training promotes social cohesion by encouraging individuals to collaborate and support their neighbors. A well-prepared community is more resilient in the face of disaster, able to organize and recover more quickly.

3. **Ensuring an effective response from emergency services**
   When citizens are familiar with emergency protocols, emergency services can respond more effectively. This reduces the burden on emergency resources and improves coordination between the various stakeholders.

Key elements of training for exceptional situations

1. **Understanding local risks**
   Every region is subject to specific risks, such as earthquakes, floods, forest fires or hurricanes. It is essential that training is tailored to the hazards specific to the geographical area concerned.

2. **Knowledge of evacuation procedures**
   Individuals must be informed of evacuation routes, assembly points and shelters available in the event of an emergency. Regular drills help to familiarize the population with these procedures.

3. **Using warning and communication systems**
   Learning to recognize warning signals, whether audible, visual or broadcast by the media, is crucial. Training should include the use of modern technologies, such as mobile alert applications, social networks and emergency messaging systems.

4. **First aid and mutual assistance**
   Teaching basic first-aid techniques enables citizens to provide assistance while waiting for help to arrive. The training also encourages mutual aid and solidarity between neighbors.

5. **Preparing an emergency kit**
   Participants should know how to prepare an emergency kit containing the essentials: water, non-perishable food, medicines, flashlights, battery-powered radios, important documents, etc.

Training adapted for maximum inclusiveness

1. **Consideration for people with disabilities**
   Training must be accessible to all, including people who are blind, deaf, have reduced mobility or cognitive impairments. This implies :

   - **Adapted teaching aids**: use of Braille, audio documents, videos with subtitles or sign language.
   - **Inclusive practical exercises**: Evacuation scenarios that take special needs into account, with adaptations for wheelchairs or guides for blind people.
   - **Trainer awareness**: Training instructors in appropriate communication and assistance techniques.

2. **Language and culture**
   It is important to adapt training content to the different languages spoken in the community and to respect cultural particularities to ensure optimal understanding and participation.

Teaching methods for effective training

1. **Interactive workshops**
   Workshops keep participants engaged by allowing them to practice the skills they have learned. They can include first aid demonstrations, evacuation simulations or emergency kit preparation exercises.

2. **Role-playing and simulations**
   Realistic role-plays help participants to experience the challenges of an emergency situation in a controlled environment. This boosts their confidence and ability to react effectively in a real crisis.

3. **Use of educational technologies**
   Mobile applications, e-learning modules and virtual reality tools can enrich the learning experience, especially for younger generations.

4. **Community involvement**
   Involving community leaders, local associations and non-governmental organizations strengthens the relevance of training and encourages wider participation.

Focus on fires

1. **Home fire prevention**
    - **Education on common causes**: Faulty electrical appliances, candles left unattended, electrical overloads.

- **Installation of smoke detectors**: The importance of functional fire alarms and regular maintenance.
- **Evacuation plans**: Draw up and practice family evacuation plans, identifying emergency exits and assembly points.

2. **Reaction in the event of fire**

- **Stop, Drop and Roll" rule**: Techniques for extinguishing flames on yourself.
- **Use of extinguishers**: Training on the different types of extinguishers and their proper use.
- **Safe evacuation**: Stay low to avoid smoke, touch door handles to detect heat, do not use elevators.

Focus on natural disasters

1. **Earthquakes**

- **Protection techniques**: Cover up under a solid table, keep away from windows, hold on tight until the shaking stops.
- **After the earthquake**: Check for injuries, avoid damaged structures, prepare for aftershocks.

2. **Flooding**

- **Advance preparation**: Know risk areas, have sandbags ready, protect important documents.
- **During flooding**: Do not cross moving water, move to higher ground, listen to instructions from authorities.

3. **Hurricanes and storms**

    - **Anticipation**: Monitor weather forecasts, reinforce structures, stock up on provisions.
    - **During the storm**: Stay indoors, away from windows, turn off non-essential electrical appliances.

4. **Forest fires**

    - **Prevention**: Don't light fires during drought periods, and observe all fire bans.
    - **Evacuation**: Follow recommended routes, prepare pets, inform relatives of your location.

Integration of lessons learned

After each training session or exercise, it is important to :

- **Assess performance**: Identify strengths and areas for improvement.
- **Update plans**: adapt procedures in line with feedback.
- **Strengthen communication**: Ensure that information flows effectively between the various stakeholders.

The role of authorities and organizations

1. **Local governments**

    - **Development of training programs**: Set up regular sessions accessible to all.
    - **Transparent communication**: Provide clear information on risks and safety measures.
    - **Support for community initiatives**: Encourage and fund local emergency preparedness projects.

2. **Emergency services**

    ◦ **Community collaboration**: Working closely with residents to understand their needs.
    ◦ **Ongoing training**: Ensure that staff are trained in the latest techniques and in the specific needs of vulnerable populations.

3. **Non-governmental organizations**

    ◦ **Educational resources**: Developing appropriate teaching aids.
    ◦ **Awareness**: Conduct campaigns to promote a safety culture.

Medical crisis management

- **Recognizing warning signs**

Medical crisis management

Medical crisis management is an essential element of public and individual health, aimed at ensuring a rapid and effective response to emergency situations that may endanger a person's life or health. The ability to recognize the **warning signs** of such crises is equally crucial, enabling early intervention, often before the situation worsens. Early intervention can not only save lives, but also prevent long-term complications. This article explores the fundamentals of medical crisis management and highlights the importance of early recognition of symptoms.

I. Understanding medical crisis management

Medical crisis management encompasses all actions taken to respond to an urgent medical situation. It involves effective coordination between healthcare professionals, emergency services, patients and sometimes the general public.

1. **Fundamental principles**

- **Rapid assessment of the situation**: As soon as a medical crisis occurs, it's essential to quickly assess the condition of the person affected. This includes assessing vital signs such as consciousness, breathing, pulse and blood pressure.

- **Prioritizing actions** : The actions to be taken must be prioritized according to the severity of the situation. For example, ensuring airway patency and blood circulation is paramount.

- **Effective communication**: Clear communication between emergency responders is crucial. This includes accurate transmission of information to the emergency service, coordination with other rescuers and communication with the patient where possible.

- **Application of established protocols**: Healthcare professionals follow standard protocols to manage medical emergencies, ensuring a systematic and efficient approach.

2. **Key management steps**

- **Emergency recognition**: Quickly identify that the situation requires urgent intervention.

- **Call emergency services**: Contact emergency services immediately for professional assistance.

- **First aid**: Provide first aid until help arrives, such as cardiopulmonary resuscitation (CPR) if necessary.

- **Transport to a care facility**: Organize safe transport to the nearest hospital.

- **Advanced medical care**: In hospital, the patient receives specialized care to treat the underlying cause of the seizure.

3. Role of healthcare professionals

Doctors, nurses and other healthcare professionals play a central role in medical crisis management:

- **Ongoing training**: They must keep their skills up to date through regular training in emergency techniques.
- **Teamwork**: Collaboration between different departments and specialties is often necessary for comprehensive care.
- **Rapid decision-making**: Emergency situations call for rapid decisions based on an accurate assessment of the situation.

II. The importance of recognizing warning signs

Early recognition of warning signs is essential to prevent a medical situation escalating into a major crisis. It allows us to intervene before symptoms worsen, offering a better chance of recovery.

1. What is a warning sign?

A warning sign is a symptom or set of symptoms that indicates a person may be on the verge of developing a serious medical condition. These signs can be subtle and varied, depending on the nature of the underlying condition.

2. Examples of warning signs for common conditions

- **Heart attack (myocardial infarction)** :
    - Chest pain or discomfort, often described as pressure or tightness.
    - Pain radiating to left arm, neck, jaw or back.
    - Shortness of breath, cold sweat, nausea or dizziness.

- **Stroke**:
    - Sudden weakness or numbness of the face, arm or leg, often on only one side of the body.
    - Difficulty speaking or understanding language.
    - Visual disturbances, severe headaches with no apparent cause, loss of balance.

- **Severe allergic reaction (anaphylaxis)** :
    - Itching, rash, swelling of the face, lips or throat.
    - Difficulty breathing, wheezing.
    - Drop in blood pressure, dizziness, loss of consciousness.

- **Hypoglycemia in diabetics**:
    - Trembling, excessive sweating, intense hunger.
    - Confusion, irritability, coordination disorders.
    - Loss of consciousness if not treated promptly.

3. The role of education and awareness-raising

- **Training the general public**: Learning to recognize warning signs enables individuals to act quickly, either for themselves or for others.

- **Awareness campaigns**: Public health institutions regularly organize campaigns to inform people about the symptoms of common medical emergencies.

- **Specific programs for people at risk**: Patients with chronic illnesses are often given detailed advice on what to look out for.

III. Strategies for improving medical crisis management

1. First aid training

- **First aid courses**: Encouraging the general public to take first aid courses, including CPR, can increase survival rates in medical emergencies.

- **Accessible training**: Offer training adapted to different groups, including children, the elderly and people with disabilities.

2. Setting up early warning systems

- **Communication technologies**: Use mobile applications or connected devices to quickly alert emergency services.

- **Automated external defibrillators (AEDs)**: Install AEDs in public places and train citizens in their use.

3. Strengthening health infrastructures

- **Rapid response times**: Improve the availability and speed of emergency medical services.

- **Inter-departmental coordination**: Facilitating communication between the various healthcare players to ensure integrated care.

IV. The role of relatives and the community

1. Family support

- **Careful observation**: Family members are often the first to notice subtle changes in their loved ones.
- **Knowing your medical history**: Being aware of existing medical conditions enables you to react appropriately.

2. Community solidarity

- **Neighborhood programs**: Set up mutual aid networks to monitor and assist vulnerable people.
- **Information sharing**: Organize workshops or meetings to discuss medical emergencies and appropriate responses.

V. Obstacles to effective medical crisis management

1. Lack of training

- **Low level of first aid training**: Many people are not trained in life-saving techniques.
- **Misinformation**: Misconceptions about medical emergencies can lead to inappropriate actions.

2. Cultural and linguistic factors

- **Language barriers**: Communication difficulties can delay the call for help.
- **Stigma**: Fear of judgment or shame can prevent some people from seeking help.

3. Limited access to care

- **Rural or isolated areas**: Response times may be longer due to remoteness.
- **Socio-economic inequalities**: disadvantaged populations may have less access to healthcare resources.

VI. Future prospects

1. Technological innovation

- **Healthcare applications**: Development of applications capable of detecting physiological anomalies and alerting emergency services.
- **Artificial intelligence**: Using AI to analyze data in real time and predict the risk of medical crises.

2. Public health policies

- **National training programs**: integrating first aid into school and university curricula.
- **Infrastructure investment**: Improving emergency services and communications networks.

- **Collaboration with emergency services**

Effective collaboration with emergency services is a fundamental pillar in the management of critical situations, whether medical, environmental or technological. Such collaboration involves close coordination between citizens, health professionals, community organizations and emergency services such as fire, police and emergency medical services. The aim is to ensure a rapid, coherent and effective response to protect the life, health and property of affected individuals and communities.

I. The importance of collaboration with emergency services

1. Fast and efficient response

Well-established collaboration reduces response times. By working in synergy, the various players can share crucial information, coordinate their actions and avoid duplication or gaps in response.

2. Resource optimization

Pooling human, material and information resources ensures optimum use of available resources. This is particularly important during major crises, when resources can be limited.

3. Continuity of care and management

Smooth collaboration ensures that victims receive continuous care, from the scene of the incident to their final destination. This includes the transfer of essential medical information for appropriate care.

4. Strengthening community resilience

By involving local communities and encouraging their active participation, collaboration with emergency services helps to strengthen people's ability to cope with and recover from crises.

II. Collaboration mechanisms

1. Effective communication

- **Clear communication channels**: Establish dedicated lines of communication between emergency services and other responders.
- **Use of modern technologies**: Integrate digital tools such as mobile applications, secure radio networks and information-sharing platforms.
- **Common language**: Adopt standardized terminology to avoid misunderstandings.

2. Shared protocols and procedures

- **Joint response plans**: Develop emergency plans that involve all relevant players.
- **Joint training**: Organize joint training sessions and exercises to strengthen coordination.
- **Regular updates**: Revise and update protocols in line with feedback and technological developments.

3. Sharing information

- **Centralized database**: Maintain a platform where relevant information can be stored and consulted in real time.
- **Confidentiality and security**: Protect sensitive data while facilitating access for authorized personnel.

- **Alerts and notifications**: Set up early warning systems to quickly inform the parties concerned.

III. Role of the various players in the collaboration

1. Emergency medical services (EMS)

- **On-site intervention**: Provide first aid, stabilize patients and decide on the most appropriate referral.
- **Coordination with hospitals**: passing on essential medical information in preparation for patient reception.
- **Participation in exercises**: Take part in simulations to improve collective preparation.

2. Firefighters

- **Fire and technical rescue management**: Responding to fires, road accidents and collapses.
- **Rescue and extrication**: Use specialized equipment to extract victims.
- **Prevention**: Raising public awareness of risks and safety measures.

3. Law enforcement

- **Securing the scene**: Ensuring the safety of intervention areas to protect responders and victims.
- **Crowd management**: Control access and prevent panic.
- **Investigation**: Gather information to determine the causes of the incident.

4. Health professionals

- **Medical care**: Offer appropriate care to victims once they arrive at health facilities.

- **Communication with EMS**: Ensure smooth transfer of information for continuity of care.
- **Participation in planning**: Collaborate on the development of emergency protocols.

5. Citizens and communities

- **First witnesses**: Provide valuable information to the emergency services.
- **First aid**: Apply first aid techniques while waiting for professionals to arrive.
- **Community involvement**: Get involved in preparedness and resilience programs.

IV. Collaboration challenges and possible solutions

1. Communication barriers

- **Challenges**: Differences in terminology, saturation of communication channels, language problems.
- **Solutions**: Training in inter-departmental communication, use of resilient communication technologies, adoption of clear, standardized language.

2. Inter-departmental coordination

- **Challenges**: Institutional rivalries, unclear roles and responsibilities, incompatible procedures.
- **Solutions**: Establish clear protocols, create coordination positions, foster a culture of collaboration.

3. Limited resources

- **Challenges**: Shortage of personnel, equipment or funding.
- **Solutions** : Sharing resources, pooling equipment, seeking joint financing.

4. Information management

- **Challenges**: Information overload, inaccurate or obsolete data.
- **Solutions**: Implementation of integrated information systems, training in data management, regular verification of information.

V. Best practices for effective collaboration

1. Joint training and regular exercises

- **Objective**: Strengthen mutual trust, improve coordination and identify weak points.
- **Implementation**: Organize realistic simulations involving all emergency services and stakeholders.

2. Setting up unified command centers

- **Objective**: Centralize decision-making and operations coordination.
- **Implementation**: Create temporary or permanent structures where representatives from different departments work together.

3. Community involvement

- **Objective**: Involve citizens in emergency preparedness and response.
- **Implementation**: Promote volunteer programs, offer first-aid training, create neighborhood networks.

4. Use of information and communication technologies

- **Objective**: Facilitate fast, secure information sharing.

- **Implementation**: Develop dedicated applications, use social media to disseminate alerts, adopt collaborative platforms.

VI. Case studies of successful collaboration

1. Natural disaster management

During a major flood, collaboration between meteorological services, local authorities, emergency services and communities enabled at-risk areas to be evacuated in good time, thus reducing human and material losses.

2. Response to a terrorist attack

In the case of an attack in an urban environment, rapid coordination between the police, emergency medical services, hospitals and municipal authorities enabled victims to be treated efficiently and the area to be made safe.

VII. Future prospects

1. Technological innovation

- **Artificial intelligence**: using AI to analyze data in real time and predict resource requirements.
- **Augmented reality**: Help responders visualize building plans or risk areas.
- **Drones and robots**: Deploying autonomous devices for reconnaissance or material delivery.

2. Comprehensive, integrated approach

- **Internationalization of protocols**: Harmonize procedures at international level to facilitate mutual assistance.
- **Taking environmental issues into account**: adapting strategies to climate change and new emerging risks.

Chapter 14

The future of care for the blind

Emerging trends in healthcare

- **Telemedicine and remote care**

Telemedicine and **remote care** represent a major revolution in healthcare, transforming the way medical services are delivered and received. Thanks to technological advances, it is now possible to provide quality care without the need for the physical presence of the patient or the healthcare professional. This development offers promising prospects for improving access to care, optimizing medical resources and meeting the current challenges facing the healthcare system.

A natural evolution of modern medicine

Telemedicine is not an entirely new concept. Its roots go back to the earliest attempts at remote medical communication, such as the use of the telegraph to transmit medical information in the XIXe century. However, it was with the advent of the internet, mobile technologies and advanced communication tools that telemedicine really took off. It encompasses a variety of services, from real-time video consultations to remote diagnostics and continuous patient monitoring via connected devices.

The undeniable advantages of telemedicine

1. **Greater accessibility to care**
   Telemedicine overcomes the geographical barriers that limit access to healthcare services. Patients living in rural or isolated areas can consult specialists without having to travel long distances. This is particularly beneficial for elderly populations or those with reduced mobility.

2. **Optimizing time and resources**
   Remote consultations reduce waiting times and unnecessary travel. Healthcare professionals can

manage their time more flexibly, resulting in greater overall efficiency in the healthcare system.

3. **Continuity of care for chronic conditions**
Patients suffering from chronic illnesses such as diabetes or hypertension benefit from regular monitoring without the need for frequent visits to the practice. Home monitoring devices transmit the necessary data to healthcare professionals in real time, enabling rapid adjustments to treatments.

4. **Responding to health emergencies**
During health crises such as the COVID-19 pandemic, telemedicine proved essential in limiting the spread of the virus while ensuring continuity of care. It helped maintain the link between patients and caregivers, despite social distancing measures.

A wide range of telemedicine applications

1. **Teleconsultation**
Teleconsultation is one of the most widespread forms of telemedicine. It enables patients to consult general practitioners or specialists via secure video calls. This makes preliminary diagnoses, prescription renewals and medical advice easier.

2. **Remote medical monitoring**
Patients wear connected devices that continuously measure vital parameters such as heart rate, blood pressure and glucose levels. This data is transmitted to healthcare professionals, who can quickly detect any abnormalities and intervene if necessary.

3. **Teleradiology**
Medical images (X-rays, scans, MRIs) are sent to remote radiologists for interpretation. This speeds up

the diagnostic process, especially in facilities where radiologists are not always available on site.

4. **Telepsychiatry**
   Mental health also benefits from telemedicine. Remote psychological or psychiatric consultations offer easier access to care, particularly for people living in areas with no specialized professionals, or for those who prefer discretion.

5. **Emergency telemedicine**
   In emergency situations, teams in the field can communicate with specialists remotely to obtain immediate advice. This is crucial for interventions in remote areas or during natural disasters.

Telemedicine challenges and considerations

Despite its many advantages, telemedicine presents challenges that must be recognized and overcome.

1. **Technological barriers**
   Not all patients have access to a reliable Internet connection or the equipment needed to benefit from telemedicine services. It is essential to develop solutions to reduce this digital divide.

2. **Data security and confidentiality**
   The transmission of sensitive medical data raises privacy concerns. Telemedicine platforms must comply with strict security standards to guarantee the confidentiality of patient information.

3. **Regulations and legal framework**
   The laws governing the practice of telemedicine vary from country to country, and can be complex. It is necessary to harmonize regulations to facilitate the

practice of healthcare professionals and protect patients' rights.

4. **The patient-caregiver relationship**
   The human relationship is at the heart of medical care. Some fear that telemedicine will reduce the quality of this interaction. It is important to preserve this dimension by developing approaches that maintain the bond of trust between patient and caregiver.

The impact of the COVID-19 pandemic

The global health crisis has accelerated the adoption of telemedicine. Faced with the need to limit physical contact, many healthcare systems rapidly integrated remote care into their routine practices. This has enabled not only immediate needs to be met, but also telemedicine tools to be tested and improved on a large scale. Feedback has been positive overall, showing satisfaction on the part of both patients and healthcare professionals.

Future prospects for telemedicine

1. **Integrating artificial intelligence**
   Artificial intelligence (AI) offers innovative possibilities for telemedicine. Machine learning algorithms can help diagnose, predict disease progression and personalize treatment. For example, applications can analyze symptoms reported by patients to guide care.

2. **Development of connected healthcare devices**
   Wearable devices such as smartwatches and implantable sensors collect a wealth of data in real time. This information enriches medical monitoring and enables more proactive medicine.

3. **Telesurgery and virtual reality**
   Telesurgery, although still in its infancy, enables

surgeons to operate remotely using surgical robots controlled via secure networks. Similarly, virtual and augmented reality offer tools for remote medical training and real-time assistance during operations.

4. **Personalized care**
   Telemedicine promotes a patient-centered approach, where care is tailored to individual needs. Patients become active players in their own health, with easier access to information and services.

- **Artificial intelligence and diagnostics**

Artificial intelligence (AI) is revolutionizing the medical field, particularly diagnostics, by offering powerful tools to detect disease with unprecedented accuracy and speed. Thanks to sophisticated algorithms and the analysis of vast quantities of data, AI is transforming the way healthcare professionals assess, diagnose and treat patients. This evolution promises not only to improve the quality of care, but also to optimize healthcare system resources.

A new era in medical diagnostics

Traditionally, medical diagnosis has relied on the expertise of doctors interpreting symptoms, medical history and test results. However, with the increasing complexity of medical data and the need for greater precision, AI is emerging as an indispensable ally. It can rapidly analyze complex information, spot subtle patterns and help clinicians make informed decisions.

AI applications in diagnostics

1. Medical image analysis

AI is particularly effective in the interpretation of medical images, such as X-rays, MRIs, CT scans and pathological images. **Deep learning algorithms**, notably convolutional neural networks, are capable of detecting anomalies with an accuracy comparable to, or even superior to, that of human experts.

For example, in breast cancer screening, AI systems analyze mammograms to identify suspicious microcalcifications or masses, enabling early detection of the disease. Similarly, in ophthalmology, AI helps diagnose diabetic retinopathy by examining images of the retina, improving the prevention of blindness in diabetic patients.

2. Predictive diagnostics and personalized medicine

AI exploits **machine learning algorithms** to analyze clinical, genomic and environmental data, in order to predict the risk of disease in individuals. In cardiology, for example, it can estimate the likelihood of a myocardial infarction based on factors such as age, lifestyle and family history.

This approach paves the way for **personalized medicine**, where treatments are tailored to the specific characteristics of each patient, improving therapeutic efficacy and reducing side effects.

3. Natural language processing and decision support

Natural language processing (NLP) techniques enable AI to analyze medical texts, such as patient records or scientific publications. This facilitates the extraction of relevant information, the monitoring of adverse drug reactions and the updating of clinical knowledge.

Intelligent virtual assistants can also provide doctors with real-time diagnostic recommendations, based on reported symptoms and available medical data.

4. Early detection of epidemics

By analyzing data from a variety of sources, such as Internet searches, social networks or electronic health records, AI can identify trends indicating the emergence of epidemics. This enables health authorities to react quickly to contain the spread of disease.

Benefits for patients and healthcare professionals

- **Greater accuracy**: AI reduces diagnostic errors by identifying subtle clinical signs that the human eye might miss.

- **Time savings**: Automated analyses speed up the diagnostic process, enabling faster patient management.

- **Improved access to care**: In remote regions or areas with low medical density, AI offers invaluable diagnostic support, filling the gap left by the lack of specialists.

- **Optimization of resources**: By automating certain tasks, healthcare professionals can concentrate on more complex aspects of care, improving the overall efficiency of the healthcare system.

Challenges and ethical considerations

Despite its benefits, the integration of AI into medical diagnostics raises important questions.

1. Reliability and clinical validation

It is essential to ensure that AI algorithms are reliable and clinically validated. Errors or biases in training data can lead to incorrect diagnoses. Rigorous validation of AI tools is therefore crucial to ensuring patient safety.

2. Transparency and explainability

AI models, particularly deep neural networks, are often perceived as "black boxes" that are difficult to interpret. It's important to develop explainable algorithms so that doctors understand the reasons behind AI recommendations, thereby boosting confidence in these systems.

3. Data protection and confidentiality

The use of AI requires access to large amounts of sensitive medical data. It is imperative to comply with data protection regulations, such as the RGPD in Europe, to guarantee the confidentiality and security of patient information.

4. Impact on the doctor-patient relationship

It is essential that the adoption of AI does not undermine the human relationship between doctor and patient. AI must be seen as a complementary tool, supporting clinical judgment rather than replacing it.

The role of the doctor in the age of AI

Artificial intelligence is not intended to replace healthcare professionals, but to assist them. Physicians continue to play a central role in interpreting AI results, making clinical decisions and communicating with patients. Their expertise is essential for integrating AI recommendations into the overall context of the patient's health, taking into account individual nuances that machines cannot always grasp.

Future prospects

The future of AI in medical diagnostics is bright, with ongoing developments that could radically transform healthcare.

- **Multimodal integration**: Future AI systems will be able to simultaneously analyze different data sources (images, text, biological signals) to provide even more accurate diagnoses.

- **Federated learning**: This approach enables algorithms to learn from decentralized data, without transferring it to a central server, thus reinforcing data confidentiality.

- **Human-machine collaboration**: The development of collaborative AI systems, where human and machine work in tandem, will maximize each other's strengths to improve clinical outcomes.

Patient participation in research

- **Expert patient groups**

Expert patient groups are an emerging and essential component of today's healthcare system. They bring together patients who, through their personal experience of illness, have acquired in-depth expertise not only on their own condition, but also on the care system, available treatments and psychosocial aspects related to their pathology. These expert patients play a key role in improving medical management, therapeutic education and the empowerment of other patients.

Origin and definition of the expert patient

The concept of the expert patient emerged in the 1990s, thanks in particular to the work of Dr. David Tuckett and the Stanford School of Medicine. The basic idea is that patients, by living with their illness on a daily basis, develop valuable knowledge and skills. They thus become active players in their own health, and can help other patients better manage their condition. An expert patient is not only informed about his or her illness, but also trained to share his or her experience in a constructive and educational way.

Roles and missions of expert patient groups

1. **Therapeutic patient education (TPE)**
   Expert patients play an active role in therapeutic education programs. Their personal experience enables them to understand the challenges faced by patients and to provide practical advice on managing the disease on a daily basis. They help translate medical information into understandable terms, facilitating treatment adherence and disease self-management.

2. **Peer support**
   Sharing experiences creates a sense of community and belonging. Expert patients offer emotional support, break isolation and help new patients overcome the psychological obstacles associated with accepting the disease. They organize discussion groups, workshops or online forums to foster exchanges and encourage solidarity.

3. **Participation in clinical research**
   By collaborating with researchers, expert patients help steer clinical studies towards questions that really matter to patients. Their involvement can improve participant recruitment, protocol design and

dissemination of results, making research more relevant and patient-centered.

4. **Improving the quality of care**
   Patient experts work closely with healthcare professionals to improve clinical practices and service organization. Their unique perspective enables them to identify weak points in the healthcare system and propose innovative solutions to remedy them.

5. **Patient advocacy**
   Expert patients play an essential role in raising public and political awareness of the issues surrounding certain diseases. By campaigning for better access to care, for the recognition of certain pathologies or for improved healthcare policies, patient experts help to change the system in favor of patients.

Training and recognition of expert patients

To become an expert patient, it's not enough to have personal experience of the disease. Specific training is often required to acquire pedagogical and communication skills, as well as an in-depth understanding of medical and psychosocial aspects. In France, universities, patient associations and healthcare institutions offer training programs that sometimes lead to recognized certification.

This training generally covers :

- **In-depth knowledge of the disease**: pathophysiology, treatments, medical follow-up.
- **Communication techniques**: active listening, group facilitation, conflict management.
- **Ethics and deontology**: confidentiality, respect for others, limits of the expert patient's role.

Institutional recognition of expert patients is growing, with increasing integration into care teams and public health projects.

Impact of expert patient groups on the healthcare system

1. **Patient empowerment**
   By sharing their knowledge and experience, expert patients help others to better understand their disease, make informed decisions and become actively involved in their care. This leads to better treatment adherence and improved quality of life.

2. **Improving the patient-caregiver relationship**
   The presence of patient experts promotes more open communication and better mutual understanding between patients and healthcare professionals. They act as a bridge between the two parties, facilitating dialogue and trust.

3. **Optimizing care paths**
   By identifying obstacles and inefficiencies in the healthcare system, patient experts help to create smoother care pathways tailored to patients' real needs. Their involvement can reduce unnecessary hospitalizations and improve coordination between the various players involved.

4. **Contributing to research and innovation**
   By participating in research projects, expert patients add value by directing work towards relevant priorities and ensuring that results are applicable in real life. They also encourage innovation by proposing new approaches based on their own experience.

Challenges and prospects

Despite the obvious benefits, integrating expert patients into the healthcare system poses certain challenges:

- **Clarifying status and role**
 It is essential to clearly define the role of expert patients to avoid confusion with healthcare professionals. This includes official recognition, conditions of practice and associated responsibilities.

- **Ongoing training**
 Expert patients must have access to ongoing training to keep up to date with medical advances and teaching techniques. This guarantees the quality and relevance of their work.

- **Ethics and confidentiality**
 Respecting the confidentiality of information and adopting an ethical stance are essential to maintaining the trust of patients and professionals alike.

- **Equity and diversity**
 It's important to ensure that expert patients represent the diversity of the population (age, gender, origin, socio-economic status) to meet the needs of all patients.

Concrete success stories

1. **Therapeutic education programs**
 In the field of diabetes, trained patient experts run workshops to help newly-diagnosed patients manage their blood sugar levels, adapt their diet and integrate physical activity into their daily lives.

2. **Participation in hospital steering committees**
 In some hospitals, expert patients sit on steering committees to contribute their perspective on the

organization of care, the quality of reception and the services offered.

3. **Participatory research**
Research projects include expert patients right from the study design stage, ensuring that the questions asked and the methods used are relevant and respectful of the participants.

4. **Advocacy and awareness-raising**
Expert patient groups have succeeded in influencing health policies, for example by obtaining recognition for certain rare diseases or changing legislation on access to innovative treatments.

- **Co-construction of care protocols**

The **co-construction of care protocols** is an innovative approach that aims to actively involve patients, healthcare professionals and other stakeholders in the development of medical protocols. This collaborative approach recognizes that patients, through their lived experience of illness, possess valuable expertise that can enrich the quality and relevance of care. By integrating the perspectives of patients, caregivers and experts, co-construction fosters more personalized, efficient and human-centered medicine.

A new vision of healthcare

Traditionally, care protocols are developed by healthcare professionals and medical experts, based on scientific data and clinical guidelines. However, this approach can overlook patients' needs, preferences and day-to-day realities. Co-construction proposes a more inclusive vision, where each stakeholder is considered a full partner in the decision-making process.

The foundations of co-construction

1. **Active patient participation**
   Patients are no longer simply recipients of care, but become active players in their own health. Their personal experience of illness, their expectations and their values are taken into account to develop protocols that truly meet their needs.

2. **Interdisciplinary collaboration**
   Co-construction involves close collaboration between different healthcare professionals: doctors, nurses, pharmacists, psychologists, social workers, etc. This multidisciplinary approach ensures that protocols are comprehensive and adapted to the various dimensions of care.

3. **Integrating scientific and empirical knowledge**
   Scientific data remains an essential foundation, but it is enriched by the empirical knowledge of patients and caregivers. This combination enables us to develop protocols that are more realistic and applicable in daily practice.

The benefits of co-construction

1. **Improved quality of care**
   By integrating patient feedback, protocols are better adapted to the realities of the field, improving their effectiveness and acceptability. Care becomes more personalized, taking into account the specific characteristics of each individual.

2. **Improved treatment adherence**
   Patients involved in protocol development are more likely to understand and accept proposed treatments. Their active participation promotes better compliance and improved clinical outcomes.

3. **Valuing the role of patients and caregivers**
   Co-construction recognizes and values the expertise of both parties. Patients feel listened to and respected, while healthcare professionals enrich their practice through a better understanding of their patients' needs.

4. **Innovation and adaptation**
   Co-constructed protocols are more flexible, and can be adjusted in line with developments in medical knowledge and feedback from the field. This adaptability fosters innovation and continuous improvement in care.

Implementing co-construction

1. **Creating mixed working groups**
   Set up teams comprising patients, healthcare professionals and, if necessary, representatives of associations or caregivers. These groups work together to identify needs, define objectives and draw up protocols.

2. **Organization of participatory workshops**
   Workshops provide an opportunity to exchange ideas, share experiences and build solutions together. They encourage everyone to express themselves and co-create content.

3. **Using facilitation methods**
   Techniques such as brainstorming, mind maps or role-playing can be used to stimulate creativity and encourage the participation of all group members.

4. **Validation and experimentation**
   Protocols are tested in the field, with careful monitoring of results and feedback. Any necessary adjustments are made to optimize their effectiveness.

5. **Training and awareness-raising**
   It is essential to train participants in the principles of co-construction and to raise their awareness of the importance of collaboration. This includes developing skills in communication, active listening and teamwork.

Examples of co-construction in practice

1. **Chronic disease management**
   In the treatment of type 2 diabetes, for example, the co-construction of protocols makes it possible to integrate patients' preferences in terms of diet, physical activity and medication follow-up. Patients share their difficulties and successes, helping to adapt recommendations to their lifestyle.

2. **Palliative care**
   At the end of life, patients and their families have specific needs and wishes. Co-constructing palliative care protocols enables us to respect patients' wishes, improve their comfort and support their loved ones.

3. **Mental health**
   In the field of psychiatry, involving patients in the development of treatment plans promotes a better understanding of their condition and greater adherence to proposed therapies.

Challenges and obstacles to overcome

1. **Cultural and organizational barriers**
   Co-construction requires a paradigm shift in the patient-caregiver relationship. Some professionals may be reluctant to share decision-making power, while patients may be reluctant to express their opinions.

2. **Managing time and resources**
   Involving patients in protocol development requires

additional time and resources. It is important to plan these activities and integrate them into the organization of care.

3. **Training participants**
   All players need to be trained in co-construction methods and the skills required to participate effectively in collaborative processes.

4. **Maintaining scientific quality**
   It is essential to strike a balance between patient preferences and scientific data. Protocols must remain evidence-based, yet tailored to individual needs.

Future prospects

The co-construction of care protocols is part of a wider trend towards participative, patient-centred medicine. In the future, this approach could be extended to other fields:

- **Use of digital technologies**
  Online platforms and mobile applications can facilitate patient participation, enabling them to share their experiences and contribute to discussions in a flexible way.

- **Participatory research**
  Involve patients right from the design stage of clinical studies to ensure that research questions are relevant and that results are applicable in real-life practice.

- **Health policies**
  Political decision-makers can integrate co-construction into the development of healthcare policies, by consulting patients and citizens to define priorities and strategic orientations.

Appendices

- **Bibliographic resources**

Here is a selection of bibliographical resources to help you delve deeper into the topics covered, such as adapted first aid, crisis communication with blind people, adapting emergency protocols, telemedicine, artificial intelligence in medicine, expert patient groups and co-construction of care protocols.

Appropriate first aid and medical crisis management

1. **"First aid guide for people with disabilities"**
   French Red Cross, 2018.
   This practical guide details first aid techniques, adapting them to the specific needs of people with disabilities.

2. **"First aid: techniques adapted to disabilities".**
   Lecomte, Alain. Éditions Maloine, 2016.
   A book that explores first aid methods adapted to different forms of disability.

3. **"Medical emergency management: principles and applications"**
   Larcan, Alain. Éditions Masson, 2015.
   A reference for understanding the fundamentals of medical emergency management.

Crisis communication with blind people

4. **"Communicating with visually impaired people in emergency situations"**
   Association Valentin Haüy, 2017.
   A guide for responders to improve communication with blind people during crises.

5. **"Accessibility and visual disability: issues and prospects"**
   Rouanet, Hélène. Presses Universitaires de France, 2016.
   An analysis of accessibility challenges for visually impaired people, including crisis situations.

Adapting emergency protocols and training to exceptional situations

6. **"Planning for and managing emergency situations: a guide for professionals"**
   Lagadec, Patrick. Éditions d'Organisation, 2014.
   A book that addresses emergency planning and management, with a focus on adapting protocols.

7. **"First aid training: integrating specific needs"**
   Ministry of the Interior, Direction Générale de la Sécurité Civile, 2019.
   An official manual for first aid training with vulnerable people in mind.

Telemedicine and remote care

8. **"Telemedicine: issues and practices"**.
   Perleth, Matthias. Éditions Elsevier Masson, 2018.
   An exploration of the various aspects of telemedicine, from its implementation to the challenges encountered.

9. **"E-health and telemedicine: innovations and prospects"**
   Bardet, Jean-Michel. Dunod, 2017.
   This book analyzes the impact of digital technologies on medical practice.

Artificial intelligence and diagnostics

10. **"Artificial intelligence in medicine: clinical applications and perspectives"**
    Davenport, Thomas H., and Dreyer, Keith. MIT Press, 2019.
    An in-depth study of AI integration in the medical field, particularly for diagnostics.

11. **"Big Data and artificial intelligence in healthcare"**
    Topol, Eric. Johns Hopkins University Press, 2019.
    The author examines how massive data and AI are transforming healthcare.

Expert patient groups and co-construction of care protocols

12. **"Expert patients: towards collaborative medicine"**
    Fleury, Muriel. Presses de l'École des Hautes Études en Santé Publique, 2016.
    A book that highlights the growing role of patients in the healthcare system.

13. **"Co-constructing care: patients and professionals together"**
    Carrick, Roxanne. Springer Publishing, 2017.
    An analysis of the methods and benefits of co-constructing care protocols.

14. **"Therapeutic patient education: concepts, aims and practices."**
    Gagnayre, Rémi, and D'Ivernois, Jean-François. Éditions Maloine, 2015.
    A guide to therapeutic education, emphasizing the partnership between patients and caregivers.

Additional resources

15. **"Universal accessibility and inclusive design"**
    Imbert, Brigitte. Éditions L'Harmattan, 2015.
    This book explores the principles of universal accessibility in various fields, including healthcare.

16. **"Inclusive first aid manual"**
    Fédération Nationale de Protection Civile, 2018.
    A practical manual for first aiders, incorporating the necessary adaptations for people with disabilities.

Websites and online resources

- **Ministry of Solidarity and Health**
  www.solidarites-sante.gouv.fr
  Official information on health policies, telemedicine and national programs.

- **French National Authority for Health (HAS)**
  www.has-sante.fr
  Recommendations, guides and reports on good medical practice and innovation in healthcare.

- **Association Valentin Haüy**
  www.avh.asso.fr
  Resources for blind and partially-sighted people, including training and advice.

- **French Red Cross**
  www.croix-rouge.fr
  First aid training, social action programs and information on accessibility.

- **French National Institute for Research in Computer Science and Control (INRIA)**
  www.inria.fr
  Research and publications on artificial intelligence applied to healthcare.

These resources provide a solid foundation for exploring topics related to adapting care, integrating new technologies into medicine and actively involving patients in their healthcare journey. They reflect the contemporary evolution towards a more inclusive, collaborative and patient-centered approach to healthcare.

- **Useful contacts and professional networks**

The care and support of blind and partially-sighted people requires close collaboration between various players: specialized associations, public bodies, healthcare professionals, educators and self-help networks. These professional contacts and networks play a crucial role in improving the quality of life of the people concerned, by offering resources, adapted services and invaluable support. Here is a list of the main organizations and networks in France working in this field.

www.ingramcontent.com/pod-product-compliance
Lightning Source LLC
Chambersburg PA
CBHW071651240526
45469CB00021B/1943